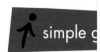

simple g

Eczema

Dr Rebecca Fox-Spencer

Dr Tim Mitchell

Eczema
First published – April 2006

Published by
CSF Medical Communications Ltd
1 Bankside, Lodge Road, Long Hanborough
Oxfordshire, OX29 8LJ, UK
T +44 (0)1993 885370 F +44 (0)1993 881868
enquiries@bestmedicine.com
www.bestmedicine.com

We are always interested in hearing from anyone
who has anything to add to our Simple Guides.
Please send your comments to *editor@csfmedical.com*.

Author Dr Rebecca Fox-Spencer
Managing Editor Dr Eleanor Bull
Medical Editor Dr Tim Mitchell
Science Editor Dr Scott Chambers
Production Editor Emma Catherall
Layout Jamie McCansh and Julie Smith
Operations Manager Julia Savory
Publisher Stephen I'Anson

Photographs on pages 16–19, 22 and 71–3
are reproduced courtesy of Dermnet.com
www.dermnet.com

ISBN-10: 1-905466-10-2
ISBN-13: 978-190546-610-8

Printed in Italy.

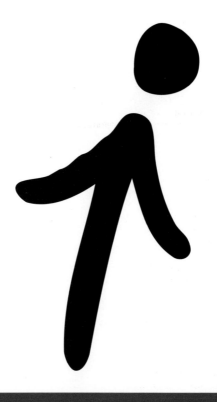

FOREWORD

TRISHA MACNAIR
Doctor and BBC Health Journalist

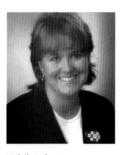 Getting involved in managing your own medical condition – or helping those you love or care for to manage theirs – is a vital step towards keeping as healthy as possible.

Whilst doctors, nurses and the rest of your healthcare team can help you with expert advice and guidance, nobody knows your body, your symptoms and what is right for *you* as well as you do.

There is no long-term (chronic) medical condition or illness that I can think of where the person concerned has absolutely no influence at all on their situation. The way you choose to live your life, from the food you eat to the exercise you take, will impact upon your disease, your well-being and how able you are to cope. You are in charge!

Being involved in making choices about your treatment helps you to feel in control of your problems, and makes sure you get the help that you really need. Research clearly shows that when people living with a chronic illness take an active role in looking after themselves, they can bring about significant improvements in their illness and vastly improve the quality of life they enjoy.

Of course, there may be occasions when you feel particularly unwell and it all seems out of your control. Yet most of the time there are plenty of things that you can do in order to reduce the negative effects that your condition can have on your life. This way you feel as good as possible and may even be able to alter the course of your condition.

So how do you gain the confidence and skills to take an active part in managing your condition, communicate with health professionals and work through sometimes worrying and emotive issues? The answer is to become better informed. Reading about your problem, talking to others who have been through similar experiences and hearing what the experts have to say will all help to build up your understanding and help you to take an active role in your own health care.

Simple Guides provide an invaluable source of help, giving you the facts that you need in order to understand the key issues and discuss them with your doctors and other professionals involved in your care. The information is presented in an accessible way but without neglecting the important details. Produced independently and under the guidance of medical experts *Eczema* is an evidence-based, balanced and up-to-date review that I hope you will find enables you to play an active part in the successful management of your condition.

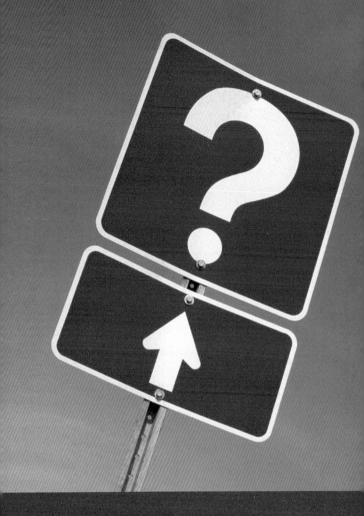

What happens normally?

WHAT HAPPENS NORMALLY?

Most of us take healthy skin for granted. After all, as long as it keeps your insides in, it's doing its job, isn't it?

Skin is very underrated. You might think that it is just there to hold your insides in, but it has plenty of other important jobs as well. Just as your heart and lungs are considered to be major organs, so is your skin.

You can give your skin credit for the following functions.

- **Protection** – your skin makes you waterproof! As well as making sure that you don't frizzle up on a hot day or swell up like a balloon when it rains, your skin protects you from bacteria, ultraviolet (UV) radiation and other nasties. Being strong and yet elastic, it also acts as a kind of shock absorber when you have a bump or fall.

- **Temperature regulation** – goose bumps and hairs sticking up when you're feeling cold? Sweating and flushed cheeks when you're hot or have a fever? Without you even thinking about it, your skin is reacting to temperature changes in your body, working to keep your body temperature just right!

The skin is the largest body organ by weight, making up about one-sixth of your total body weight.

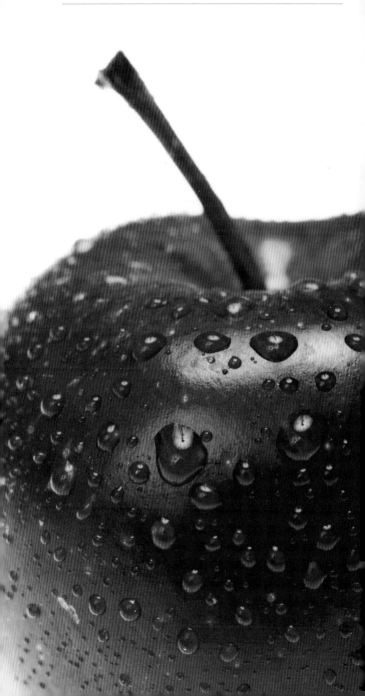

- **Interaction with your environment** – your skin is your point of contact with the outside world. Receptors in your skin, which are linked to your brain via nerve cells, enable you to feel the difference between rough tree bark and a polished table top, or between sandpaper and silk. They also allow you to feel pain, which is crucial for your own protection. For example, if you burn your hand on a hot oven door, you will automatically pull it away, preventing more serious damage.

- **Making vitamin D** – vitamins are naturally-occurring substances which are necessary for the proper growth and functioning of the body. Vitamin D has many important functions, but people tend to get very little of it from the food in their diets. Vitamin D can be made by the skin with the help of UV light found in the sun's rays, and this is the most important source of the vitamin for most of us.

- **Storing calories** – the skin contains a very fatty layer which is important for reducing heat loss from the body. This layer also stores calories, in a 'reserve' supply which can be tapped into when you are not getting enough calories from your diet.

- **Physical appearance** – the condition of our skin is often a reflection of our general health and well-being. For those of us who are not fortunate enough to have nice clear skin, concerns about physical appearance can have a major impact on our self-esteem. The decoration of the skin, with make-up, jewellery, tattoos or paints can be important both socially and culturally in different ethnic groups.

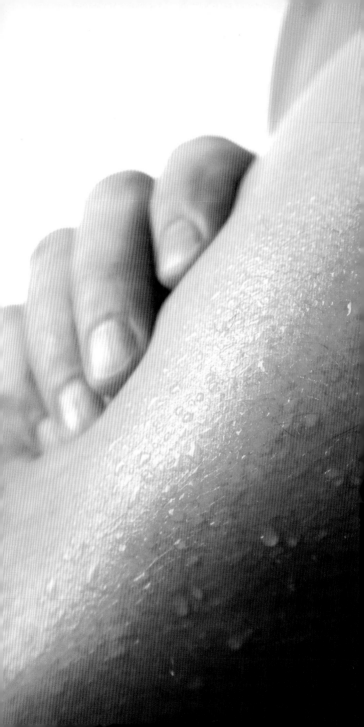

THE STRUCTURE OF SKIN

Your skin is clearly not just an oddly shaped piece of stretchy fabric. It has a complicated structure with many different components. There are three basic layers in your skin.

1. **The epidermis** – the outermost layer of the skin. In this layer, skin cells are held together by fatty substances called lipids, a bit like the way in which bricks are held together by cement. Skin cells in the epidermis are constantly being replaced. They multiply deep in the epidermis, and are pushed up towards the surface as newer ones are generated beneath them. The cells become flatter, tougher and more waterproof as they approach the surface of the skin. Once there, skin cells flake off naturally from the surface of the skin. The epidermis needs to be made up of at least 10–15% water for it to function as a flexible and effective barrier. Any less water than this and the skin will be dry and prone to cracking.

2. **The dermis** – the layer underneath the epidermis, composed of tough collagen and stretchy, elastic fibres. The main role of the dermis is to sustain and support the epidermis, by providing oxygen and nutrients and taking away waste products. It also takes the brunt of the body's knocks and bumps, and gives the skin its ability to regulate temperature and feel touch and pain.

3. **The subcutaneous layer** – the deepest layer, rich in insulating fat cells.

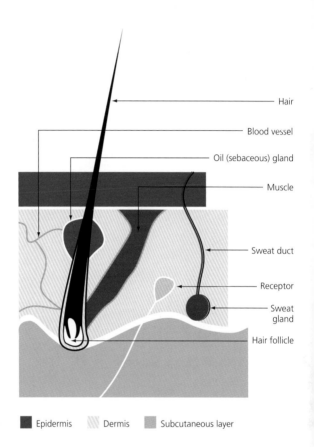

Hair

Blood vessel

Oil (sebaceous) gland

Muscle

Sweat duct

Receptor

Sweat gland

Hair follicle

■ Epidermis   ░ Dermis   ■ Subcutaneous layer

**OUR SKIN HAS THREE BASIC LAYERS:
THE EPIDERMIS, THE DERMIS AND
THE SUBCUTANEOUS LAYER.**

Within these three layers are a number of structures.

- **Glands** – sweat glands embedded in the dermis produce sweat, which is taken to the surface of the skin through sweat ducts. Oil (sebaceous) glands release an oily substance called sebum directly onto the epidermis. This helps to keep the skin supple.

- **Blood vessels** – tiny blood vessels supply the skin with oxygen and nutrients, and remove unwanted waste products.

- **Receptors** – these allow us to feel touch and pain as well as sensing the outside temperature.

- **Hairs** – project from a follicle deep in the skin to the outside world. By standing up, they can trap an insulating layer of air around your body to bring your body temperature up. By lying flat, they allow heat to be lost through the skin to the surrounding air.

PUTTING SKIN TO THE TEST

Even people who consider themselves to have healthy skin will find that it reacts if it is challenged, such as in the case of sunburn or bee stings, for example. Often, and in both of these cases, a skin reaction involves inflammation. Although sunburn can cause other more serious and long-term problems (such as an increase in the risk of certain skin cancers), these cases of inflammation are temporary and should resolve without the need for any further treatment.

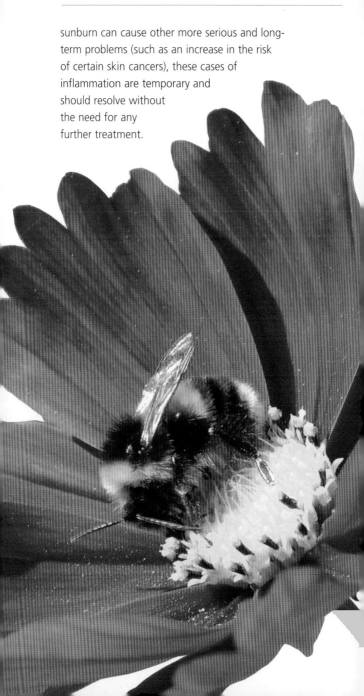

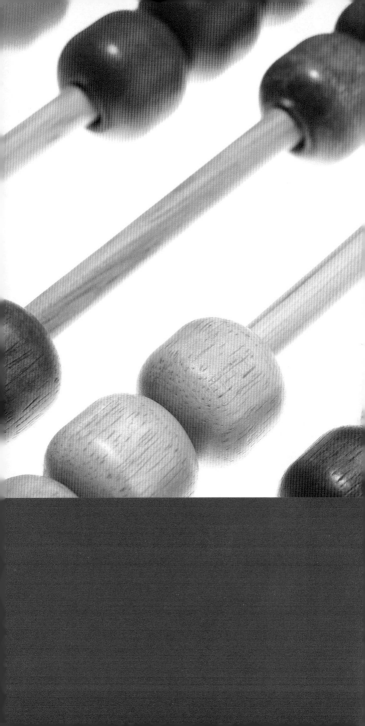

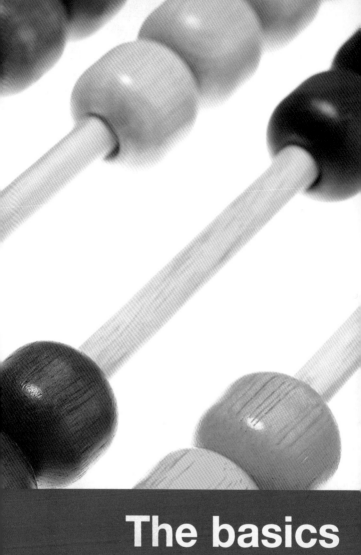

The basics

ECZEMA – THE BASICS

There is a lot we still don't know about eczema. Having an understanding of what we do know, though, can help you to manage your condition and limit the impact that it has on your life.

WHAT IS ECZEMA?

Eczema, also sometimes called 'dermatitis', is a disorder of the skin which is characterised by intense itch (technically known as pruritus) and inflammation (as seen in sunburn or nettle stings). When skin is affected by eczema, it is not the smooth, supple protective barrier that it should be. People with eczema frequently have dry skin which is susceptible to developing bacterial, viral or fungal infections. Patches of skin affected by eczema will probably be red, often with lumps or blisters.

ECZEMA AND DERMATITIS

People often use the terms eczema and dermatitis interchangeably. However, dermatitis is a more general term than eczema, and literally means inflammation of the skin. In the past, dermatitis has been used to describe skin inflammation which is brought on by known triggers outside the body, whereas eczema was used when the condition had no known cause. To avoid confusion, we will refer to eczema, rather than dermatitis, throughout this book.

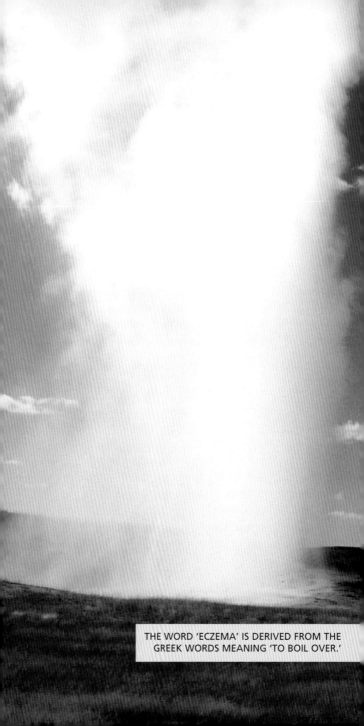

THE WORD 'ECZEMA' IS DERIVED FROM THE GREEK WORDS MEANING 'TO BOIL OVER.'

THE DIFFERENT TYPES OF ECZEMA

Atopic eczema

Atopic eczema is the most common form of eczema, and will be the main focus of this book. A person who has atopy, or is atopic, has a tendency to develop allergies. Being atopic means that your immune system does not develop as it should, and you are more likely to become sensitive to external factors in the environment that a non-atopic person would not react to. When the immune cells in your skin react inappropriately to something in the environment, it can result in the skin becoming red and inflamed (a bit like a nettle sting). This is called a hypersensitivity reaction.

Who gets it?

Most people who are diagnosed with eczema in the UK have atopic eczema. Many people with atopic eczema also have asthma and/or allergic rhinitis (of which hay fever is the 'seasonal' form), which are also atopic conditions.

In the vast majority of cases, atopic eczema develops during childhood. It is quite common in schoolchildren in the UK, with roughly one-in-six showing some symptoms of eczema. Five per cent of adults in the UK suffer from atopic eczema and new cases rarely develop during adulthood.

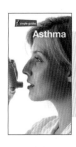

For more information see
Asthma

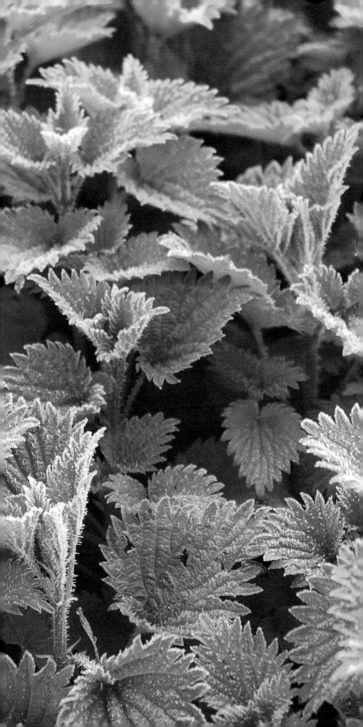

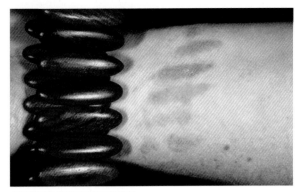

ALLERGIC CONTACT ECZEMA

ALLERGIC CONTACT ECZEMA

What is it?

This type of eczema occurs when the skin comes
into contact with a substance to which a person
has become allergic (called an allergen), for
example certain metals such as nickel in jewellery,
or fragranced products such as perfume or soap.
Some people might also become allergic to foods
that they handle, such as fish. The skin reaction
usually occurs locally at the point where contact
with the allergen occurred.

Who gets it?

In many cases, allergic contact eczema occurs in
people who also suffer from general atopic eczema.
They may even have become sensitive to some of
the ingredients in creams or lotions which they are
using to control the symptoms of atopic eczema.
Nickel jewellery and some types of perfume can
also cause allergic contact eczema.

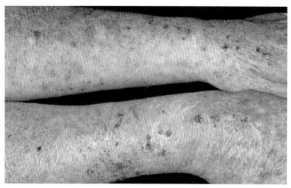

IRRITANT CONTACT ECZEMA

IRRITANT CONTACT ECZEMA

What is it?

This occurs when the skin comes into contact with irritating substances such as the chemicals found in certain domestic cleaning agents. Irritant contact eczema is much more common than allergic contact eczema. Given that our hands are the most likely part of our bodies to come into contact with irritants, they are the most common area to be affected by irritant contact eczema.

Who gets it?

Irritant contact eczema may occur in anyone exposed to irritant substances – there is no allergy involved. Common irritants include bleach and other cleaning agents, paint and adhesives. Certain occupations (e.g. cleaning) and hobbies (e.g. DIY) can put you at an increased risk of this form of eczema. Prolonged exposure to water can cause the cells in the skin to swell, and weaken the protective barrier. Thus, irritant contact eczema is particularly common in people who have to get their hands wet frequently, like hairdressers, food handlers, doctors and nurses.

DISCOID ECZEMA

What is it?

Discoid eczema appears as round patches of eczema (hence the term discoid) on otherwise normal skin, although it can also occur in people who have atopic eczema. Often the patches are found in a symmetrical position on the limbs.

Who gets it?

Discoid eczema can affect people of all ages, but is particularly common in middle-aged or elderly men.

SEBORRHOEIC ECZEMA

What is it?

This can sometimes look like a mild dandruff problem, but when it is more severe, it can cause redness and scaling on other parts of the body. It most often appears on the scalp, on the face, in skin creases such as the groin and armpits and, in small children, around the nappy area. It can be caused by a yeast infection.

DISCOID ECZEMA

SEBORRHOEIC ECZEMA

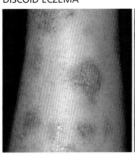
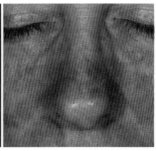

Who gets it?

Seborrhoeic eczema can occur at any stage of adulthood, most commonly in men, though a particular form of the condition affects babies in their first year of life.

VARICOSE ECZEMA

What is it?

This affects the lower legs and ankles. It occurs when there are problems with the circulation, such that blood is not being pumped upwards out of the legs as effectively as it should be.

Who gets it?

Varicose eczema generally occurs in middle-to-late adulthood, and particularly in women and those who are overweight. Anybody with circulatory problems, such as those with chronic heart disease, previous deep vein thrombosis (DVT) or varicose veins, is at increased risk of varicose eczema.

VARICOSE ECZEMA

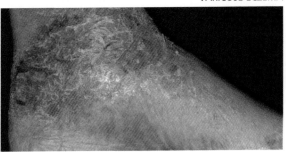

THE SYMPTOMS OF ATOPIC ECZEMA

The main symptoms of atopic eczema are:

- itch – this is the characteristic symptom: if it doesn't itch, it's not atopic eczema
- redness
- dry, cracking and scaling skin
- blisters
- skin thickening
- oozing and crusting skin.

There are different 'hot spots' on the body where eczema is most likely to prove a problem, though these will vary depending on your age and race. In infants, patches of eczema occur most frequently on the face, but as they get older, their arms and legs are more likely to be affected. In particular, in Caucasian children, the backs of the knees and the insides of the elbows might be affected. In black or Asian children, the fronts of the knees and outside points of the elbows are more susceptible. People who continue to experience eczema into adulthood may start to develop more patches on their face again.

Where the surface of the skin is broken, it becomes more susceptible to infection. If skin is infected, it might ooze clear fluid from burst blisters. When the oozing fluid dries, it can leave yellowish crusts of protein on the skin. The infection can spread to other regions of affected skin, particularly if the infectious agent (bacteria, virus or fungal spores) is rubbed around the skin whilst applying creams and other products.

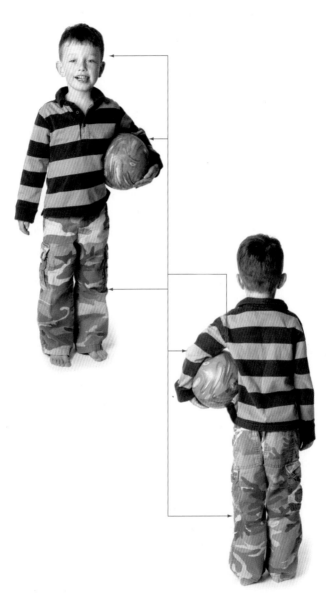

THE ARE 'HOT SPOTS' ON THE BODY WHERE ECZEMA
MAY PROVE TO BE A PROBLEM.

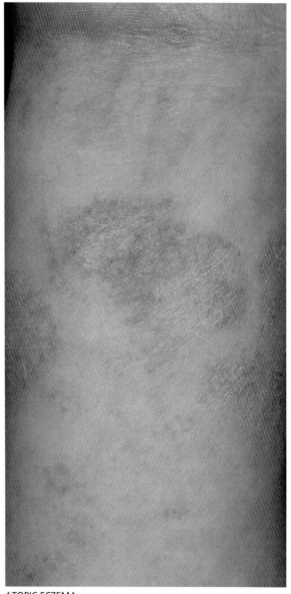

ATOPIC ECZEMA

THE BURDEN OF ATOPIC ECZEMA

Atopic eczema is not just a case of having a bit of an itch now and again. It can have a serious impact on the quality of peoples' lives, many of whom, of course, are children. The 'burden of eczema' can include the following.

- **Physical discomfort** – due to intense itch and the wounds that result from scratching.

- **Disruption of sleep** – itching during the night can wake you, and indeed the people who sleep near you.

- **Disruption at work or school** – distraction caused by itching and the need to apply creams and lotions frequently can disrupt your working day. Eczema may also restrict your ability to do certain types of job (e.g. working with animals or jobs that involve regular contact with water).

- **Psychological impact** – having red, sore, itchy patches on the skin, and in some cases open wounds resulting from scratching, can be hugely damaging to a person's self-esteem.

- **Cost** – the cost of buying medications, skin conditioning products and protective clothing, and the time and inconvenience of regularly applying them, may be a problem for some people.

CAUSES AND TRIGGERS OF ATOPIC ECZEMA

If you have eczema, the reasons that you developed it in the first place may never become totally clear. You may have inherited a susceptibility to becoming atopic from your parents. There is also a theory that atopy is more likely to develop in people who were exposed to a very sterile environment in childhood – we will explore this so-called 'hygiene hypothesis' in more detail later (see *Why me?* page 36).

Certain factors may cause your eczema to flare up. If you have atopic eczema, your symptoms may worsen when you are exposed to certain allergens (substances to which you are allergic). Common allergens include:

- the skin and faeces of house-dust mites
- animal dander
- mould
- certain foods (e.g. milk, nuts)
- pollen.

Your eczema may also flare up more easily in response to contact with irritants, as the barrier function of the skin is not so strong. These irritants, to which you are not allergic, may include:

- certain fabrics
- soaps, cosmetics, perfumes
- detergents and other cleaning fluids
- water.

Some people report that emotional stress can also make their eczema symptoms flare up.

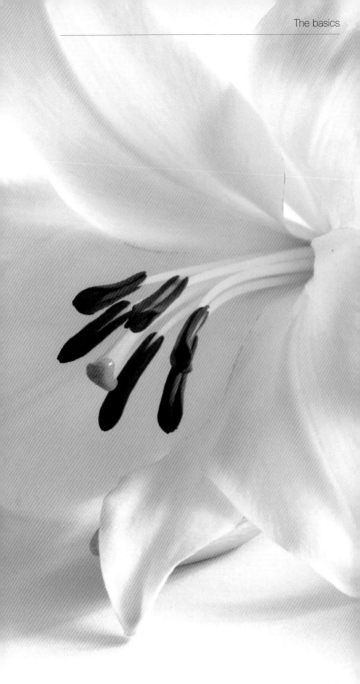

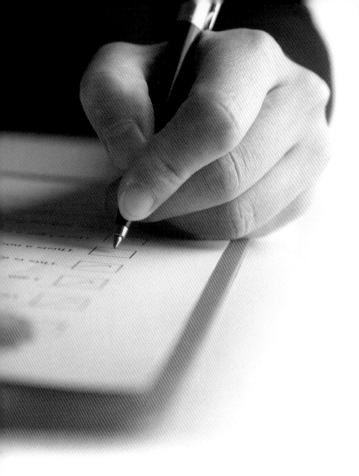

WHEN TO SEEK MEDICAL HELP

If you, or your child, have dry, itchy skin and
believe that it could be eczema, it is important to
consult your GP. Approximately 15% of the UK
population visit their doctor with a skin condition
each year, and eczema accounts for nearly a third
of these complaints.

Your GP will be able to diagnose the condition
and, although they cannot cure your eczema,
there are effective treatments which they can
prescribe for you.

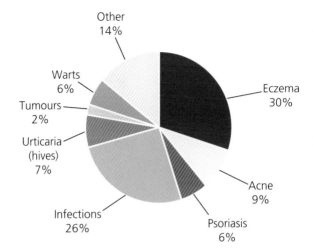

**FREQUENCY OF SKIN DISEASES SEEN BY GPS
IN THE UK** *www.abpi.org.uk*

DIAGNOSING ECZEMA

If you go to your doctor because you suspect that
you might have eczema, he or she will carry out a
physical examination, as well as asking you about
signs of eczema or other atopic conditions in your
own or your family's past. Eczema might be
suggested by a number of factors:

- itchy skin (if it doesn't itch, it is very unlikely to
  be eczema)
- the presence of other atopic conditions
  (e.g. asthma, allergic rhinitis)
- general dry skin
- symptoms starting in early childhood.

Your doctor may also ask about how the condition
affects your everyday life, and will need to know
exactly what treatments you are using, even if they
are just moisturisers or herbal remedies.

27

MANAGING ECZEMA

Eczema can be a huge burden to the person it affects and, if they are a child, their parents too. However, there is an extensive range of products available to help prevent and control eczema flare ups.

Skin care

- Use of moisturisers/emollients (an emollient is a mixture of oils, fats and water).
- Care for the skin during and after bathing.
- Avoidance of clothes that are itchy and scratchy.
- Guarding against irritants by wearing protective clothing (e.g. gloves).
- General avoidance of allergens and irritants.
- Adoption of a healthy diet.

Treatments available from your doctor

- Emollients
- Topical corticosteroids
- Topical immunomodulators
- Antimicrobials
- Antihistamines

Treatments available from a skin specialist (dermatologist)

- Systemic immunosuppressants
- Phototherapy

Treatments you can try yourself

- Probiotics
- Evening primrose oil
- Oatmeal

Complementary therapy

- Chinese herbal medicine
- Reflexology
- Homeopathy
- Acupuncture
- Hypnotherapy

We will look at the various management options in more detail in *Managing eczema*.

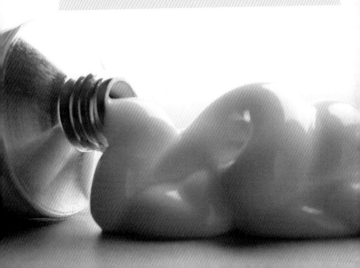

YOUR HEALTHCARE TEAM

You should work closely with your doctor to ensure that your eczema is managed as well as it possibly can be. However, it is important to be aware that eczema requires day-to-day care, and you have the ultimate responsibility for keeping it at bay. If you devote a little time each day to making sure that your skin is well cared for, you can minimise the risk of flare ups and the extent to which you will need drugs to treat them.

As well as your GP, there are other healthcare professionals who may become involved in looking after you and your eczema:

- a dermatologist

- a dermatology nurse

- a dietitian or allergy specialist

- a counsellor

- a complementary therapist.

By working with your healthcare team, you should be able to develop a routine of skin care and treatments which keeps your eczema at bay.

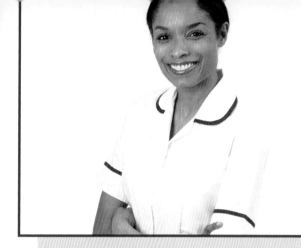

DERMATOLOGY NURSE

As a nurse who specialises in dermatology, I have a number of possible roles in the management of your eczema. Traditionally, I am based in the dermatology department of a hospital, where I provide support for the dermatologist and may run clinics. In the hospital, I can carry out certain practical aspects of your treatment, such as administering phototherapy or performing a patch test. Clinics provide you, as a patient, with the opportunity to ask questions about the practicalities of your care – how best to use your creams, how to apply wet wrapping bandages and suchlike. I will generally have time to discuss with you the lifestyle changes that might help you or your child to deal with eczema.

As well as having a base at the hospital, I can also work at a community health centre or a GP's surgery. My job is becoming increasingly important in the day-to-day management of eczema, and I now have the authority to prescribe certain medications.

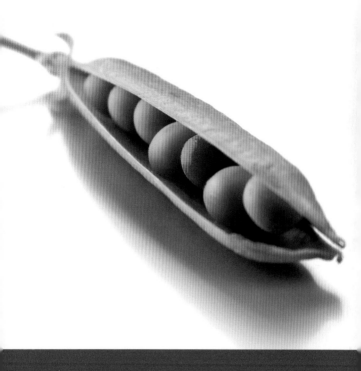

Why me?

WHY ME?

You may be wondering why you have developed eczema, particularly if it has started later in life. Alternatively, if your child has been diagnosed, you may be concerned that it has arisen because of something that you have done wrong. It is important to realise that it is not your fault.

HOW COMMON IS ECZEMA?

If you have been diagnosed with eczema, you are certainly not alone! Atopic eczema is the most common form of eczema, and is thought to affect over 2% of the UK population – that's about 1.3 million people, and this number is rising. It is about twice as common in children as it is in adults. One-in-five children in the UK has atopic eczema. Approximately 65% of people with eczema first developed symptoms before they were 1 year old, and 90% before they reached the age of 5. There does not appear to be any real effect of gender – boys are just as likely to get it as girls.

Generally, atopic eczema tends to be more common amongst people of higher social class than those of lower socioeconomic classes. Related to this, it is also more common amongst children with few siblings than those who belong to large families. There is also a certain amount of regional variation in the UK, with eczema more common in the South-East and the Midlands than in places like Scotland and Wales.

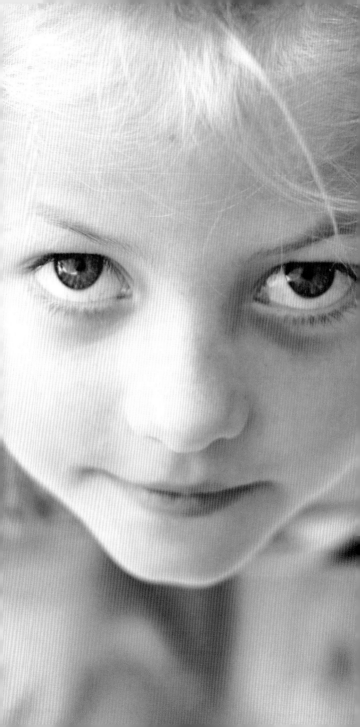

WHY IS ECZEMA BECOMING MORE COMMON?

The proportion of people in the UK affected by atopic eczema has increased by up to five times in the last 30 years, but nobody really knows why. The best accepted reason behind this surge in atopic eczema is the increased exposure to allergens. In the UK, we now heat our houses to warmer temperatures and ventilate them less. We also spend much more time indoors than we used to. This means that our exposure to house-dust mites and moulds, which thrive in these warm and moist conditions, will have increased as a result. There is now also a huge range of cleaning agents, detergents and solvents available for use in the home, which are all potential causes of contact eczema.

The hygiene hypothesis

You may have read headlines in the papers claiming that children brought up on farms are less likely to develop eczema, or that 'friendly bacteria' can be used to protect against it. These observations relate to the so-called 'hygiene hypothesis', the idea that childhood infections protect us from developing atopic conditions. In countries such as the UK, childhood infections of the gut and lung (such as typhoid fever or tuberculosis) are now rare. According to the hygiene hypothesis, this has directly resulted in more children developing allergies than ever before.

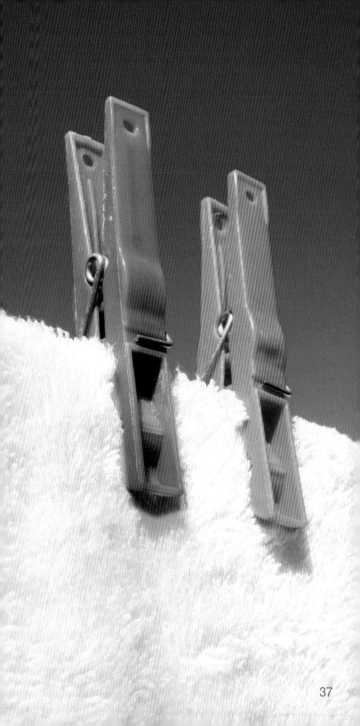

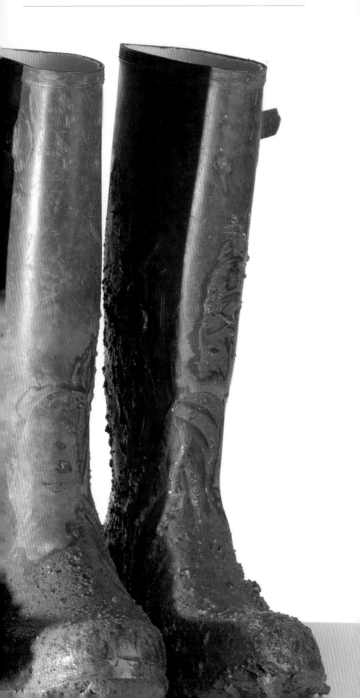

Much of the work done so far on the hygiene hypothesis has focused on the link between childhood infections and asthma, rather than atopic eczema. There is a good scientific basis for the idea that infection can trigger changes in a child's immune system which make it less likely to react inappropriately to potential allergens in the future. In other words, the child is less likely to become atopic. Exposure to infection in childhood could therefore potentially reduce the risk of asthma, atopic eczema and allergic rhinitis. The case for the hygiene hypothesis in atopic eczema is not yet as strong as it is for asthma. Scientists have shown, however, that injecting certain dead parasites under the skin can significantly improve symptoms of atopic eczema in affected children.

We are a long way from using worms to treat eczema! The hygiene hypothesis is certainly worth exploring, though. It would help to explain why children in larger families are less likely to develop eczema (due to the passing on of infections between siblings). It is also consistent with the fact that children in big cities are more likely to develop eczema than those in rural areas – not only are there more pollutant allergens in the cities (e.g. soot, diesel fumes), but children in rural areas are more likely to be exposed to infections, due to more outdoor play and exposure to livestock.

We might not be sure yet just how important the hygiene hypothesis is in eczema, but many doctors would probably already agree that lots of outdoor play and the odd mud pie or two is very conducive to a healthy childhood!

CAN OTHER PEOPLE CATCH MY ECZEMA?

It is important to understand that, even if your skin becomes infected, your eczema is not contagious. Children in particular may shy away from a friend with eczema, and it is important that the affected child knows that they cannot spread their eczema, even by contact. On the contrary, they should be encouraged to play and interact normally with other children, in order to minimise any effects that eczema might have on their self-esteem and future social skills.

HOW DID I GET ECZEMA?

Nobody knows exactly what causes eczema. Similar to other atopic conditions (asthma and allergic rhinitis), atopic eczema is thought to develop after two things have happened:

1. you inherit an increased risk for atopic conditions in your genes
2. you are exposed to substances to which you become allergic.

Although an allergy to a particular type of food might be a factor in your eczema, it is not true to say that eczema is caused by diet. In other words, allergies won't have caused your eczema, but the same genes which made you atopic will also have made you more likely to develop food allergies. Having said that, food allergy is very rare except in some children whose eczema usually started when they were less than 12 months old. Eczema usually has many different triggers so even if a suspect food is identified, it may make no difference.

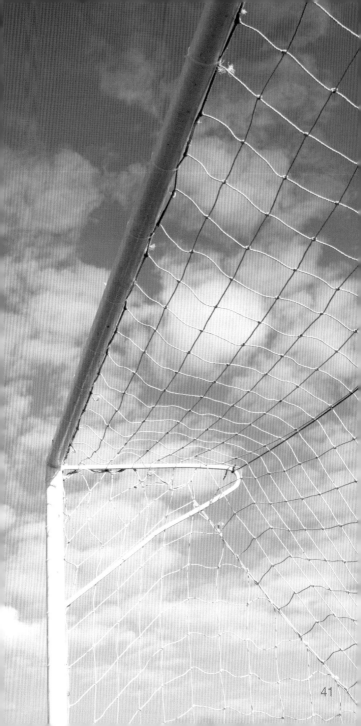

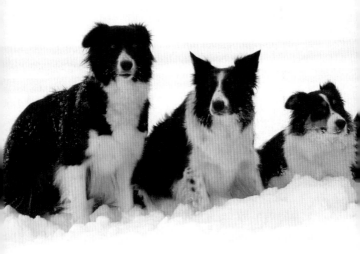

HOW WILL MY ECZEMA AFFECT MY FAMILY?

As far as your family is concerned, your eczema can be distressing for them as well as you. If you have a child with eczema, you will be well aware of how upsetting it can be to see them scratching their skin excessively and losing sleep because of the discomfort. On the other hand, the person with eczema may sleep through their scratching, and it may be the people sleeping nearby who are woken by the noise and restlessness of an itchy, scratchy person! Other children in the family can also feel neglected as decision-making often revolves around the child with eczema (like choosing types of family holidays).

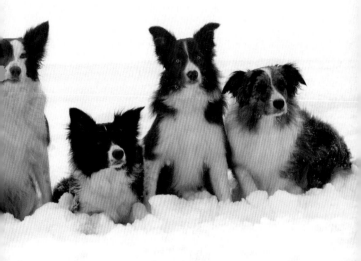

If you are a parent of a child with eczema, it is important that you receive support from your doctor, and are not left to deal with managing the eczema on your own. Make sure that you involve your GP on a regular basis so that he or she can suggest alternative approaches if you feel like you are not getting the desired results.

If you yourself are affected, remember that friends and family who do not suffer from the condition may find it very hard to understand what you are going through. They may not be able to appreciate the intensity of itch or level of discomfort that you feel, and may be frustrated with you when you can't resist the urge to scratch.

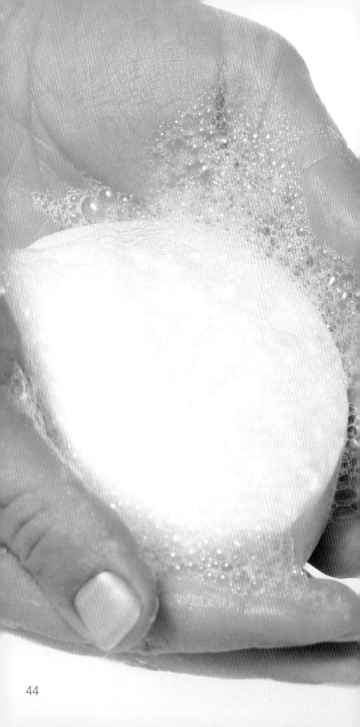

ECZEMA IN THE WORKPLACE

Not only can eczema be a burden at work, but
many aspects of your working environment can
actually make it worse. Contact eczema is the
most common kind of work-related skin condition.
Triggers for eczema in the workplace can include:

- frequent hand washing – paper hand towels
  may irritate the skin, hot air driers may dry the
  skin excessively

- soaps – especially those containing colours
  and perfumes

- air conditioning – can be very drying to
  the skin

- dust – a common allergen, can collect on
  computer screens or paperwork

- stress – can make eczema worse, and is
  arguably more likely to occur at work than
  at home

- cleaning fluids and solvents

- animal dander – a common allergen, which is
  hard to avoid if you work with animals.

Where an industrial irritant is involved, your
employer is legally obliged to protect you against
any hazard. You are also obliged to make use of
any protective measures offered to you. Apart
from this, as far as is practical, you need to try and
avoid allergens at work and apply emollients
regularly. Wear hypoallergenic gloves to protect
your hands from contact with irritants or allergens,
and to reduce the frequency of hand washing.

ECZEMA AT SCHOOL

For a young child trying to fit in at school, having patches of eczema which are impossible to cover up can be a huge burden. Other children may use it as an excuse to bully the affected child, or isolate them if they believe that the condition is infectious. If you are the parent of a child with eczema, it is important that you inform the school and agree a healthcare plan in advance of them starting school or nursery. Many of the problems at school can be alleviated simply through education, of teachers and children alike. The teacher should be made aware that the child will need to apply emollients regularly, and may need assistance in doing so. They should also be considerate of a child's unwillingness to partake in PE lessons, for example.

Simple measures like not sitting the child near to a sunny window or by a radiator can prevent the child from feeling hot and start scratching. The other children should also be made aware of what having eczema means. Activity packs for teachers are available from The National Eczema Society.

Eczema can also be particularly distressing for those who continue to suffer into their teenage years. As children begin to place more importance on their physical appearance, having visible eczema and perhaps having skin which is sensitive to shaving, or certain kinds of make-up or perfume, for example, can be very traumatic. The stresses associated with trying to be both popular and successful at school can make things worse. Teenagers should be encouraged to think positively about their condition. Encourage them to go shopping for clothes, whilst explaining the need to avoid rough fibres or irritating wool. Help them to pick out hypoallergenic skin products and make sure they know which kinds of food they need to avoid when they are out. Also, if you think they might be sexually active, it is a good idea to warn them about the possibility that they may be allergic to latex condoms.

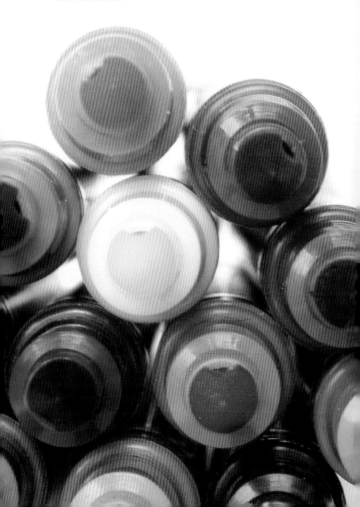

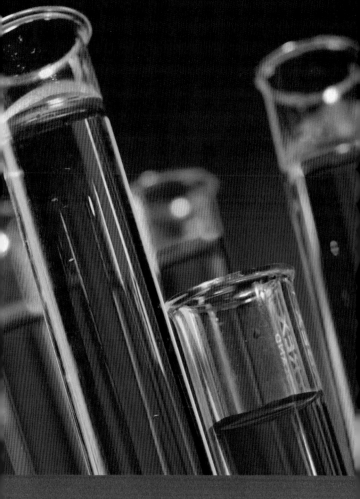

Simple
science

SIMPLE SCIENCE

In order for you to understand how the various treatments for eczema work in different situations, it will be useful for you to learn a little more about what exactly is going on in your skin when you have the condition.

DRY SKIN

As we have seen, the skin is made up of three main layers – the epidermis, the dermis and the subcutaneous layer. When we're talking about the problems in eczema, it is the epidermis, closest to the surface of the skin, which takes centre stage.

The epidermis is very thin. Even where it needs to be most robust, for example on the palms of your hands and the soles of your feet it is less than 1 mm thick. On your eyelids, it is ten-times thinner! Nonetheless, the epidermis is itself made up of a number of distinct layers of skin cells.

In the two lower layers of the epidermis (called the basal layer and the spinous layer), the cells are held together by little protein bridges. Cells in the next layer (called the granular layer), release fatty, waxy substances called lipids into the spaces between the cells of the top layer, the cornified layer. If you imagine that the cells of the cornified layer are like bricks in a wall, the lipids between the cells act as the mortar, bonding the cells together and making sure that the cornified layer acts as an effective barrier. Importantly, it means that water does not escape from the skin or seep in from outside. At least 15% of the contents of the cells of the cornified layer should be water, which enables the skin to be nicely elastic and soft.

If you have eczema, the 'lipid cement' between the cells in the cornified layer does not form properly. This means that the waterproof barrier is not effective, and water is lost from the cells in the cornified layer. The layer becomes less pliable, and cracks can form between the cells. To you, this will appear as dry skin, and because the barrier is not complete, your skin will be much more prone to irritation and infection. Importantly, soap, washing-up liquid and other detergents can remove lipids from the cornified layer and make the problem worse.

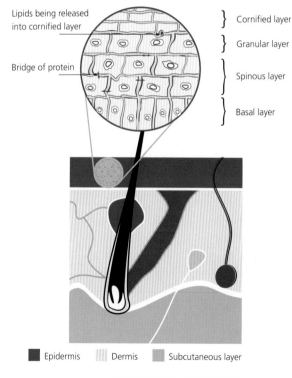

Lipids being released into cornified layer

Bridge of protein

Cornified layer

Granular layer

Spinous layer

Basal layer

Epidermis   Dermis   Subcutaneous layer

THE STRUCTURE OF THE SKIN.

Treating dry skin

Emollients (e.g. E45®, Oilatum®) are moisturising creams, lotions, ointments, bath oils and soap substitutes. They are used widely in the treatment of eczema because they help to restore the water content of dry skin by repairing the 'brick wall' structure in the cornified layer. They do this in two main ways:

- by forming an extra oily barrier over the surface of the skin which reduces water loss from the cornified layer

- by penetrating into the cornified layer and filling the gaps between the skin cells, thereby substituting for the lost lipids.

INFLAMMATION

You can have dry skin without having eczema. The problem with having cracks in the cornified layer is that irritants can penetrate the damaged barrier and enter the skin. The presence of these foreign invaders triggers a reaction by the body's immune system. Proteins called antibodies detect the foreign invaders and bind to them. By doing this, they act a bit like flags to the rest of the immune system, marking the targets which need to be destroyed. These flags attract white blood cells to the scene. These can be thought of as inflammatory cells, as they release chemical substances called histamine, cytokines and leukotrienes that cause the skin to become inflamed. Inflammation occurs because the amount of blood flow to the affected area increases, and the blood vessels which carry it become leaky, so that fluid collects between the cells and pushes them apart. Because of these effects, the skin appears red and can feel puffy and spongy.

Sometimes, it is not just the infected area of the body, but eczema all over the body, that flares up. This can happen when the *staphylococcus* bacterium is the irritant in question. In the case of irritant contact eczema, this immune reaction might be triggered by a strong detergent or glue, for example. If you are an 'atopic' person, you are more likely to develop antibodies, and therefore have inflammatory reactions, to things (e.g. house-dust mites, some foods) that other people would not be sensitive to.

Although your skin can be itchy without being inflamed, the chemicals which are released by the white blood cells, particularly histamine, promote itch.

Treating inflammation

Most of the creams that your doctor can offer you on prescription for treating eczema work by directly reducing inflammation in your skin.

- **Topical corticosteroids** (sometimes just called steroids, e.g. hydrocortisone, betamethasone esters) have been used to treat eczema for the past 40 years. They tone down the inflammatory response, by interacting with the DNA in your skin cells, thereby preventing too many 'inflammatory proteins' being made.

- **Topical immunomodulators** (tacrolimus and pimecrolimus) have only recently become available for the treatment of eczema. When applied to the skin, they reduce the activity of an enzyme (a protein which speeds up chemical reactions) which would otherwise perpetuate inflammation.

- **Systemic immunomodulators** (e.g. ciclosporin) act in the same way as topical immunomodulators, but are taken as tablets. Because they are swallowed, they exert their effects throughout the body, and thus have the potential to cause more side-effects. Some corticosteroids can also be given systemically (in tablet form) to treat eczema flare ups.

- **Phototherapy**, whereby the skin is treated with controlled exposure to UV light, is another treatment option for eczema. Although it is not entirely clear how phototherapy works, experts believe that it may have anti-inflammatory properties. One form of UV light, UVA, might be able to kill off cells which cause inflammation.

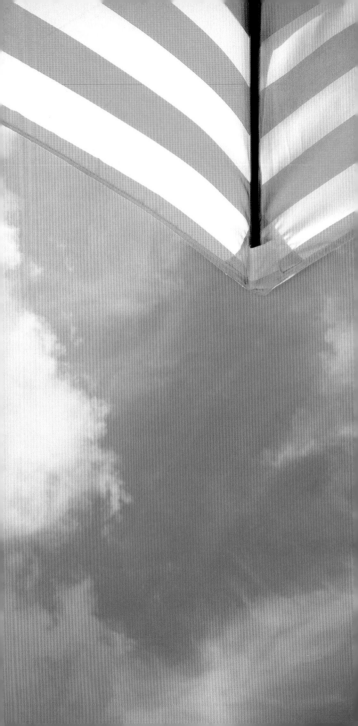

ITCHING

The itching associated with eczema can be incredibly intense, and most people with eczema would probably describe it as their most unpleasant symptom. Skin experts still don't understand itch completely. As we saw earlier, though, chemical mediators such as histamine that are involved in causing inflammation in the skin, can promote itch.

Treating itch

You have probably heard of **antihistamines** being used to treat other atopic conditions, such as allergic rhinitis. They can be used in eczema too, for reducing itch. They are not always very effective in this role, however, and some of their value lies in their sedative properties, particularly those of the older antihistamines.

Although newer drugs are generally 'non-drowsy', the older ones do cause drowsiness and so can help some people with eczema to sleep through their itch. Other treatments for reducing itch are classified as **antipruritics**, and include crotamiton, which works simply by producing a cooling effect as it evaporates from the skin.

ITCHY AND SCRATCHY?

If you are the parent of a child with eczema, no
doubt you will have looked on in horror at the relief
your itchy child seems to get from scratching their
skin raw. The pain that follows intense scratching
appears to override the sensation of itch.
Unfortunately, excessive scratching causes further
damage to the skin, worsening the eczema and
making it even more itchy. This is known as the
itch–scratch cycle.

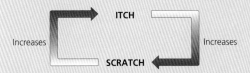

THE 'ITCH–SCRATCH' CYCLE

Experts used to believe that the sensations of both
pain and itch were communicated to the brain by the
same nerve cells. The theory was that pain could
commandeer these channels of communication, thus
blocking transmission of the itch signal. It now
appears that there are nerve cells dedicated entirely to
transmitting 'I am itchy' signals from the skin to the
brain, and that the process whereby pain overrides
the itchy feeling may happen once both the itch and
pain messages have actually reached the brain.

INFECTION

As we have already seen, the broken barrier caused by a lack of lipids in the cornified layer results in the skin becoming more susceptible to allergens and irritants. Cracking also leaves it vulnerable to infection, most often by bacteria. The most common infections associated with eczema are:

- *Staphylococcus aureus* (bacterium)

- *Streptococcus* (bacterium)

- *Herpes simplex* (virus)

- *Molluscum contagiosum* (virus)

- warts (virus)

- fungal infections.

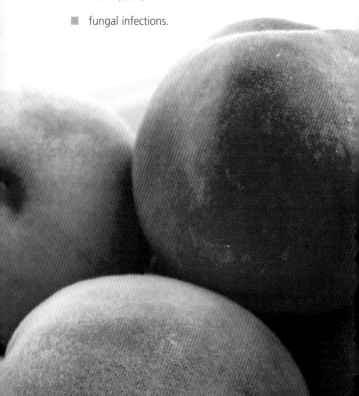

Treating infections

Because of these complications, **antibacterial** (e.g. fusidic acid), **antiviral** (e.g. aciclovir) and **antifungal** (e.g. miconazole) creams are sometimes added to standard eczema medications to treat infected skin. Some of these are available mixed together with corticosteroids (e.g. with hydrocortisone, in Fucidin H® or Daktacort® or with clobetasone butyrate, in Trimovate®) or emollients (e.g. Dermol®). There is some debate about how effective antibacterial drugs can be when administered on the skin, so the doctor might prescribe antibiotic tablets (e.g. flucloxacillin, erythromycin) instead if it is clear that your skin is infected.

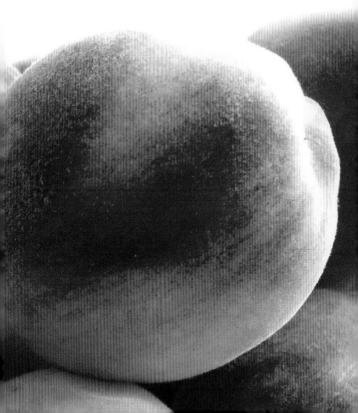

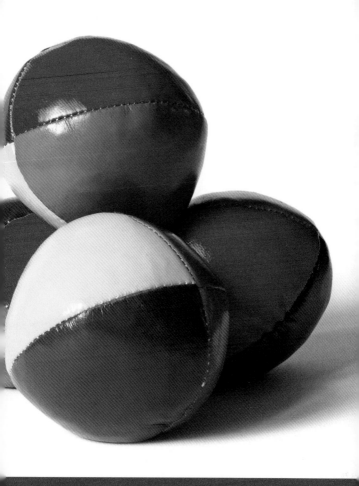

Managing
eczema

MANAGING ECZEMA

Eczema can take its toll on both your physical and your mental well-being, but this impact can be vastly reduced if the condition is managed properly. This will require some time and effort on your own part, but it is important to recognise the importance of looking after your skin properly.

HOW WILL ECZEMA AFFECT ME?

As we have seen, uncontrolled eczema can be a huge burden for somebody who is affected by it, and in the case of an affected child, for their parents too. But the good news? There is plenty that you and your doctor can do about it! There is a vast range of products available to help control the symptoms, both those which need to be prescribed by your doctor, and general skin care products which you can buy independently.

Eczema is not one of those conditions where you can blindly take a pill each day, prescribed by your doctor, without having any understanding or sense of control of your own. You are in the driving seat with eczema. You will need to work with your doctor to find the best strategy for controlling your condition, and devote some time each day to doing your bit.

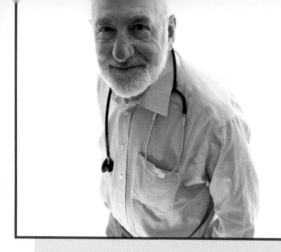

GP

As a GP, I will probably be your first port of call. My role is to recognise and diagnose your skin condition and to start the management process. This can mean prescribing medication as well as offering advice, reassurance and further explanation if you should require it. I will ask you about your symptoms and do a physical examination in order to make an accurate diagnosis.

If I feel that it is warranted, I can call on specialist opinions from a hospital dermatologist, allergist or dietitian or refer you to an eczema clinic. Once your condition and treatments are stabilised, I will work with other members of the healthcare team to ensure that regular reviews and check-ups are arranged for you. These are designed to detect and treat any changes in your eczema, good or bad, and ensure that you get the best possible care.

My overall aim is to tailor the management process to suit your individual circumstances. Developing and maintaining long-term relationships with my patients and their families helps me to do this.

WHEN SHOULD I SEE THE DOCTOR?

As we have already seen, an estimated 15% of the population consult their GP because of skin problems each year, and eczema is the most common of these. All of the following are good reasons for going to see your doctor:

- You don't yet have a diagnosis, but you have dry, itchy skin and suspect that you might have some form of eczema.

- You have already been diagnosed with eczema and prescribed treatment, but you are experiencing flare ups which are not controlled by your current medication.

- You are concerned for any reason about the treatments that you are taking and want to change the way you manage your eczema (it is important not to do this without discussing with your doctor first).

- You think that you may have identified a specific trigger for your symptoms, for example, a type of food (bear in mind, though, that food allergies are not as common as many people believe).

Most cases of eczema can be managed by you and your GP. However, he or she may feel that it is a good idea to refer you to a specialist (a dermatologist). There is no reason to be alarmed by this – you are not being palmed off as a hopeless case! Your GP will still be involved in looking after you, and you are simply adding an extra level of expertise to your care team. Possible reasons for referral to a dermatologist include:

- your eczema is not responding to the treatments your GP is offering you

- your eczema is getting worse and needing increasingly potent treatments

- there is evidence that your treatments are actually making the eczema worse

- it is appropriate for you to be tested for sensitivity to specific allergens.

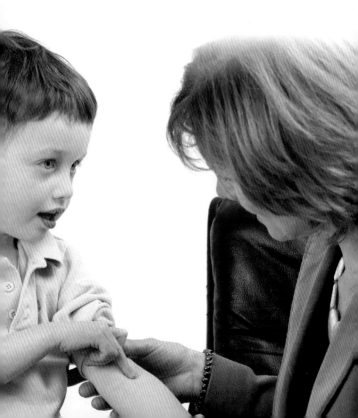

MANAGEMENT GUIDELINES

In order to make sure that doctors are aware of the most up-to-date treatments and strategies available for treating eczema and other conditions, independent bodies generate management guidelines. The main source of management guidelines in the UK is the National Institute for Health and Clinical Excellence (NICE), and specific guidelines for the management of atopic eczema have also been produced jointly by the Primary Care Dermatology Society (PCDS) and the British Association of Dermatologists (BAD).

DIAGNOSING ECZEMA

The guidelines for the management of atopic eczema produced by the PCDS and BAD advise a doctor to diagnose a person with eczema if they have an itchy skin condition (in a child, scratching or rubbing of the skin can give this away) together with at least three of the following features:

- a history of itchiness around areas where the skin creases (e.g. behind the knees, on the neck)

- a history of asthma or allergic rhinitis. If the person is under 4 years old, they need not have shown a history of atopic disease themselves – asthma, allergic rhinitis or eczema in a close relative is sufficient

- general dry skin over the previous year

- current visible eczema in the skin creases (or the face and limbs in young children)

- a history of symptoms starting before the age of 2 years.

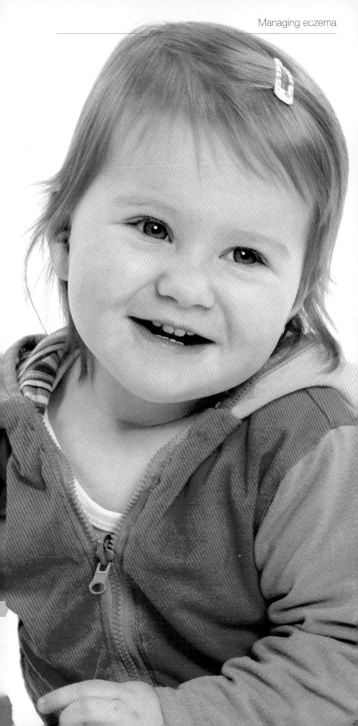

If you go to your doctor because you suspect that you have eczema, he or she will use a number of approaches to confirm a diagnosis of eczema. Similarly, if you have had eczema for some time, the doctor will need to assess whether or not to change your treatment strategy. Your doctor might:

- ask about your own symptom history, including when the problem started

- ask whether any of your close relatives have asthma, allergic rhinitis or eczema

- ask if you are aware of any specific triggers that make your symptoms get worse

- ask what treatments you are currently using or have used in the past

- ask about the impact that the symptoms have on your daily life and how they make you feel

- ask what you expect treatment to do for you

- look for evidence of infection

- assess growth (in the case of children with long-term severe eczema). This is due to a potential side-effect of one of the drug treatments for eczema in young children.

There is no specific test for eczema – you can't get a simple 'yes or no' diagnosis by using a blood or urine test. Getting through all of the questions that your doctor may want to ask you might take some time. It may take more than one appointment before you settle on a diagnosis and a plan for how you are going to tackle your eczema.

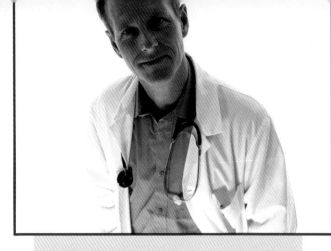

DERMATOLOGIST

I am a hospital doctor specially trained to manage conditions affecting the skin. If you have eczema, you might be referred to me by your GP. This might happen for a number of reasons: your eczema might be proving difficult to treat, or your GP might think that you are a good candidate for a particular kind of treatment that is only available from a specialist, such as phototherapy.

Some of the newer and more potent drugs for eczema can only be initiated by a dermatologist or a GP with a specialist interest in skin conditions. Also, if you and your GP think that a particular substance in your diet or environment is making your eczema worse, I can arrange for allergy testing to be carried out. Eczema can often be infected, and in some cases (such as if the skin is infected with the Herpes Simplex virus), your GP will refer you to me straight away. I will communicate directly with your GP, and we will work together to control your eczema.

WHAT ELSE COULD IT BE?

There are a number of skin conditions that have symptoms similar to those of eczema, and could be mistaken for eczema by you, or perhaps even your doctor.

Psoriasis

Psoriasis involves inflammation and can lead to thickened skin. It occurs when the rate of production of new cells in the epidermis is too high, leading to lots of underdeveloped cells being pushed onto the surface of the skin. There are a number of different forms of psoriasis.

- Plaque psoriasis – the most common form, appears as patches of raised red skin, with a well-defined edge and silvery scales on the surface.

- Nail psoriasis – tiny pits appear on the nails, and the nail may separate from the nail bed.

- Guttate psoriasis – appears mainly on the body. Usually follows a sore throat.

- Flexural psoriasis – patches are smooth and shiny, and appear in skin creases.

- Palmoplantar psoriasis – appears as blisters on the palms of the hands and soles of the feet.

- Scalp psoriasis – dry and flaky scalp, which may become red and inflamed.

- Erythrodermic psoriasis – affects the whole body.

Psoriasis most often affects people in their teens or twenties and those in their sixties, and there is some evidence that you can inherit an increased risk of developing psoriasis from your parents. There is also a strong association between psoriasis and stress levels.

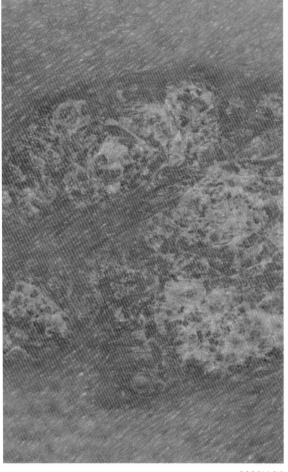

PSORIASIS

Fungal infection

Although fungal infection can occur as a complication of eczema, it can also be a problem in people who don't have eczema at all. The most common form of fungal infection is ringworm. This appears as scaly red patches which can be up to several centimetres in diameter. The skin in the middle of these patches may be quite normal – it is only the edge of the area which is affected, as the infection spreads outwards from the centre. Because skin diseases like eczema tend to be symmetrical, if the rash only occurs on one leg and not both, then it is usually an infection.

There are various forms of ringworm (technically called *tinea*), defined by the region of the body they affect:

- *Tinea corporis* – affects the 'trunk' of the body, but is sometimes used to refer to all kinds of ringworm.
- *Tinea pedis* – affects the feet (also known as athlete's foot).
- *Tinea manuum* – affects the hands.
- *Tinea capitis* – affects the scalp.
- *Tinea cruris* – affects the groin.
- *Tinea facialis* – affects the face.

FUNGAL INFECTION

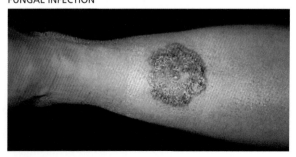

Scabies

Scabies is an itchy skin condition caused by a mite, called *Sarcoptes scabiei*. This mite burrows into the skin, and can trigger an allergic reaction which causes itching and a rash of raised, red spots. The condition is easily passed on from person to person through close contact.

Impetigo

Impetigo is caused when bacteria get into the skin through a small break in the epidermis (people with eczema are particularly at risk of this condition). It develops into blisters which spread over the skin, usually in the region of the face. These blisters are caused by infection with bacteria, and impetigo is highly contagious. It most commonly affects children and teenagers, with nurseries and playgroups at particular risk of being affected due to a high rate of transmission between young children, probably as a result of close physical contact.

SCABIES

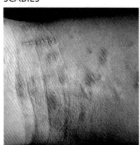

IMPETIGO

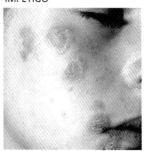

SKIN CARE

A major underlying problem in eczema is the lack of moisture in the skin. As we saw in the *Simple science* section, the lotions, creams and ointments that are collectively known as emollients can help to restore moisture levels in the skin. The different types of emollient vary in how easy they are to spread over your skin and how effective they are as a barrier. This is because they vary in terms of their lipid content (remember, lipids are the fatty substances that are lacking in the epidermis of skin with eczema).

Therefore, choosing which kind of emollient to use often depends on which skin type you have in the affected area.

Don't be afraid to ask your doctor or pharmacist for advice on which might be a good product to try. You need to be happy with your emollient because you will need to use plenty of it!

RECOMMENDED EMOLLIENTS FOR DIFFERENT SKIN TYPES

Skin type	Lotion	Cream	Ointment
Mild skin dryness	✓	✓	
Moderate-to-severe skin dryness		✓	✓
Hairy skin	✓		
Weeping, infected eczema	✓	✓	

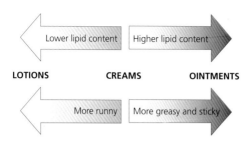

Five tips when using your emollient.

1. Don't worry that you are using too much emollient – there is no active ingredient which you can overdose on. Use it liberally on all affected areas.

2. Try to apply the emollient at least 2–3 times each day.

3. Make sure you apply emollient after bathing, washing your hands and swimming.

4. Mix and match different emollients for different purposes – you might like to use an ointment before you go to bed but a less messy cream during the daytime.

5. Don't stop using emollients if your skin clears up – keep going and reduce the risk of future flare ups.

THE EMOLLIENTS CURRENTLY AVAILABLE IN THE UK

Emollient	Lotion	Cream	Ointment
Alpha Keri Bath®			
Aquadrate®		U	
Aqueous Cream, BP		*	
Aveeno®	*	*	
Balneum®			
Balneum® Plus		U	
Calmurid®		U	
Cetraben®		*	
Decubal® Clinic		*	
Dermalo®			
Dermamist®			
Dermasalve®		*	
Dermol®	M	M	
Diprobase®		*	*
Diprobath®			
Doublebase®			
Drapolene®		*	
E45®	*	*	
E45® Itch Relief Cream		U	
Emollient Medicinal Bath Oil			
Emulsiderm®			
Emulsifying Ointment, BP			*
Epaderm®			*
Eucerin®	U	U	
Gammaderm®		*	
Hewletts®ª		*	
Hydromol®		*	*
Hydromol Emollient®			
Hydrous Ointment, BP			*
Imuderm®			
Kamillosan®			*
Keri®	*		
LactiCare®	*		
Liquid and White Soft Paraffin Ointment, NPF		*	
Lipobase®		*	
Neutrogena® Dermatological Cream		*	
Nutraplus®		U	
Oilatum®		*	
Oilatum® Plus			
Paraffin, White Soft, BP			
Paraffin, Yellow Soft, BP			
Ultrabase®		*	
Unguentum M®		*	
Vaseline Dermacare®	*	*	
Zerobase®		*	

U contains urea
M contains antimicrobials to fight infection
BP, British Pharmacopoeia
ªContains peanut oil.

Bath oil/ additive	Spray	Gel	Soap substitute	Jelly	Shower emollient
*					
*					
*					
*					
*					
*					
	*				
M					M
*					
		*			
*			*		
*					
M					
*					
*					
*					*
M					
				*	
				*	

Emollient or moisturiser

People often question whether there is any difference between an emollient and a moisturiser. The two names are often used to mean the same thing, but technically, an emollient is any substance which softens or smoothes the skin, whereas the term 'moisturiser' specifically implies adding or retaining water. One way that a moisturiser can do this is through the inclusion of a humectant, which is something that attracts water.

In practice, many products marketed as emollients contain humectants, most commonly urea. However, products which are described as moisturisers are usually intended more as beauty products for people with dry, but not eczematous skin. These often contain perfumes and other additives to make them more cosmetically acceptable. If you have eczema, it is worth bearing in mind that your sensitive skin may react to these ingredients.

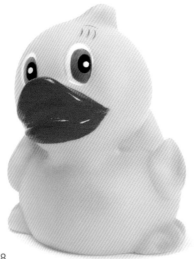
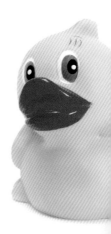

Bathing

Bathing can be a problem if you have eczema. Evaporation of water from the skin after a bath can be drying and hot water can sometimes irritate the skin further. There is some evidence to suggest that hard water (the hardness of domestic water supplies varies between regions in the UK) is worse for skin with eczema, as is water that contains high levels of chlorine. Crucially, conventional soap can be very drying, as it removes some of the already depleted 'lipid cement' from between the cells near the surface of the epidermis. The following can improve matters when taking a bath:

- don't make the bath too hot
- limit the bath to no more than 15 minutes
- use emollient bath oils and soap substitutes
- consider treating bath water to remove chlorine (using a dechlorinating filter, for example)
- pat the skin dry after bathing, instead of rubbing
- apply generous quantities of emollient immediately after drying.

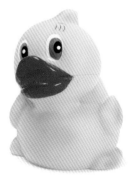
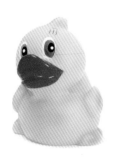
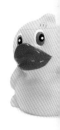

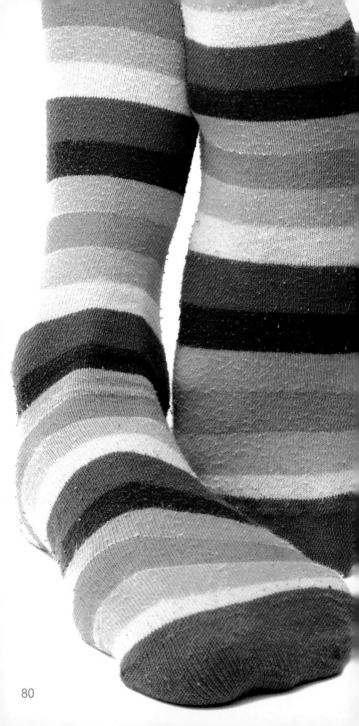

Protecting your skin against scratching

It is very easy for someone who has not suffered the intense itch associated with eczema to tell you to just ignore it. Yet anyone who has eczema can probably vouch for the fact that it is not always possible to ignore the itch. This can be a particular problem for very young children who are too young to understand why they shouldn't scratch. Even older children and adults who know that scratching will damage the skin and make the eczema worse will sometimes succumb to the itch and may also scratch in their sleep whilst they are unaware of it. Aside from treating the eczema with emollients and drugs (we will look at these later), there are a number of practical measures that may help to prevent scratching or minimise its effects:

- wear gloves, socks and/or stretchy bandages at night to offer a barrier to scratching

- cut nails short

- choose clothes and bed linen that is soft and made out of cotton, not rough, scratchy fibres

- for young children, distraction, with toys perhaps, is sometimes effective.

AVOIDING THE THINGS THAT TRIGGER YOUR ECZEMA

As we have seen, several forms of eczema involve the skin being sensitive to irritants or allergens. If you are aware of substances that trigger your eczema to get worse, avoiding these as much as is possible is obviously going to benefit your skin. It will not be practical to completely avoid irritants and allergens, but you can probably limit your exposure somewhat.

Most people with eczema will find that their symptoms become worse if they sweat, whether it be during exercise or whilst sleeping. It may be worth avoiding exercise which makes you particularly sweaty for an extended period of time, and ensure that you use cool, cotton bedclothes to avoid getting too hot at night.

Common irritants	Common allergens
Soap	House-dust mites
Washing powder	Animal dander
Cleaning fluids, solvents	Pollen
Wool	Metals (e.g. in jewellery)
Cigarette smoke	Cosmetics, perfume
Chlorine	Rubber, latex

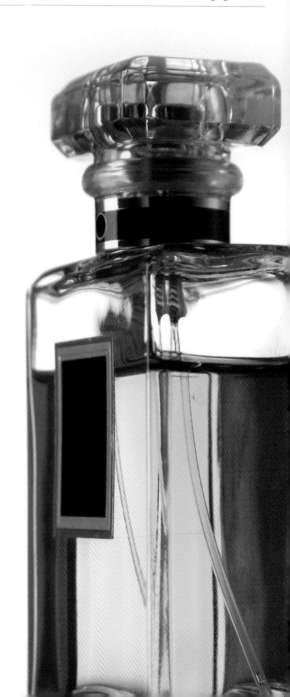

TREATMENTS AVAILABLE FROM YOUR DOCTOR

There are many drugs available for the treatment of eczema, and your doctor is best placed to decide which ones are the most appropriate for you. The choice will depend on factors such as the severity of your eczema, the regions of your body that are affected, whether or not your skin is infected and how your eczema has responded to treatments in the past.

Topical corticosteroids

Topical corticosteroids, sometimes referred to just as steroids, are the most commonly prescribed drugs for eczema. 'Topical' simply means that they are applied to the surface of the skin.

Corticosteroids are available in various strengths (or potencies), and your doctor will aim to keep your eczema controlled using the weakest drug that is effective. He or she will also advise you on how long you should use the treatment for – this is likely to be no more than 6 weeks or so. This is because the more potent the drug and the longer it is used, the higher the risk of side-effects.

TOPICAL CORTICOSTEROIDS AVAILABLE FOR TREATING ECZEMA

Potency	Topical corticosteroid	Brand name(s)
Mild	Hydrocortisone	Canesten HC®M, Daktacort®M, Dermacort®, Dioderm®, Econacort®M, Efcortalan®, Eurax Hc®C, Fucidin H®M, Hc45®, Lanacort®, Mildison®, Nystaform-HC®M, Timodine®M, Vioform-Hydrocortisone®M, Zenoxone®
	Fluocinolone acetonide	Synalar 1 in 10 Dilution®
Moderate	Alclometasone dipropionate	Modrasone®
	Betamethasone valerate	Betnovate-RD®
	Clobetasone butyrate	Eumovate®, Trimovate®M
	Fludroxycortide	Haelan®
	Fluocinolone acetonide	Synalar 1 in 4 Dilution®
	Fluocortolone	Ultralanum Plain®
	Hydrocortisone	Alphaderm®U, Calmurid HC®U
Potent	Beclometasone dipropionate	Propaderm®
	Betamethasone valerate	Betacap®, Betnovate®, Betnovate-C®M, Betnovate-N®M, Bettamousse®, Diprosone®, Diprosalic®S, FuciBET®M, Lotriderm®M
	Diflucortolone valerate	Nerisone®
	Fluocinolone acetonide	Synalar®, Synalar C®M, Synalar N®M
	Fluocinonide	Metosyn®
	Fluprednidene acetate	Acorvio® PlusM
	Fluticasone propionate	Cutivate®
	Hydrocortisone butyrate	Locoid®, Locoid Crelo®, Locoid C®M
	Mometasone furoate	Elocon®
	Triamcinolone acetonide	Aureocort®M, Tri-Adcortyl®M
Very potent	Clobetasol propionate	Dermovate®, Dermovate-NN®M
	Diflucortolone valerate	Nerisone Forte®
	Halcinonide	Halciderm Topical®

Mcontains antimicrobials
Ccontains crotamiton
Ucontains urea
Scontains salicylic acid

People are often concerned about using steroids because they associate them with the anabolic steroids used by some body-builders and athletes. Corticosteroids are very different to anabolic steroids, and are safe when used as directed by your doctor. Do not be afraid to speak to your doctor, though, if you have concerns about the side-effects or safety of the corticosteroids that you are prescribed. It is better to do this than to stop using them without voicing your concerns.

Your doctor will be monitoring you for side-effects if you are using corticosteroids. The most likely side-effects include:

- thinning of the skin
- appearance of fine lines or thin visible blood vessels on the skin
- discolouration of the skin
- triggering or worsening of other conditions like acne.

When you apply a corticosteroid to your skin, a tiny amount of the drug gets into your bloodstream. There is a very small risk that, in young children, this may stunt growth. For this reason, the doctor will monitor the growth of a child who is receiving more potent corticosteroids.

As is the case for emollients, topical corticosteroids are available in different formulations (lotions, creams, ointments, scalp applications and gels), and the choice of which to use depends on factors such as the region of skin affected, the severity of the eczema and the time of day it is to be applied. Apart from hydrocortisone and clobetasone (e.g. Hc45®),

corticosteroids are only available on prescription.
Some corticosteroids are available as compound
preparations, in which they are mixed with
antimicrobial drugs (to fight infection), crotamiton
(an anti-itch ingredient), urea (a humectant, to
attract water) or salicylic acid (which helps the
scales on the surface of the skin to separate off).

If eczema covers a large proportion of the
body and is severe, your doctor may consider
prescribing a course of oral corticosteroids
(e.g. prednisolone). These are corticosteroids in
tablet form.

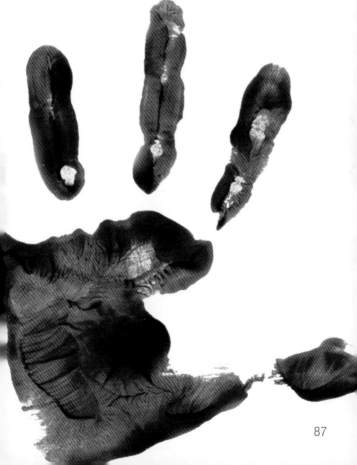

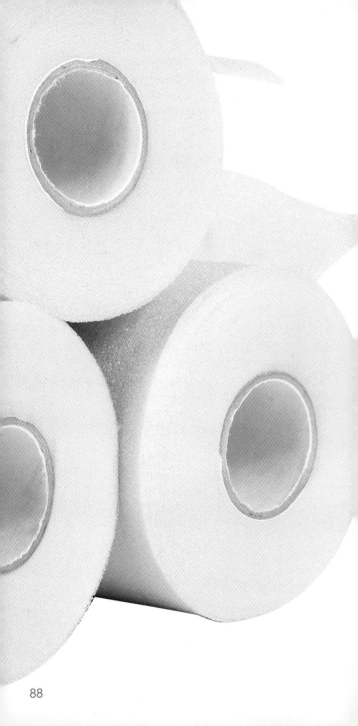

One final point about corticosteroids. Covering them up once they are applied increases their potency. In some cases, your doctor will ask you to do this on purpose (such as when you are 'wet wrapping', see below). It could be dangerous to cover up corticosteroids in an uncontrolled way, though, particularly if they are very potent. This is what will happen if you apply emollients straight after your corticosteroids. It is a good idea to try and wait half an hour after putting corticosteroids on your skin before then applying emollients to the same area.

WET WRAPPING

Wet wrapping is a technique used more often in children than in adults, and is particularly suitable for those who suffer with extreme itchiness at night and loss of sleep. It involves putting a warm, wet tubular bandage over the skin where emollients and/or topical corticosteroids have been applied. A second, dry, bandage is then put on over the top of the first. This is usually done in the evening, before going to bed. Wet wrapping serves three main purposes.

1. It permits slow evaporation of moisture from the wet bandage which thereby cools and soothes sore skin.

2. It allows topical corticosteroids to be absorbed into the skin more effectively.

3. It provides a barrier to protect the skin from scratching.

Speak to your doctor if you think that wet wrapping might help you or your child – do not attempt it without your doctor's agreement and guidance.

Topical immunomodulators

This is the most recent class of treatments to be introduced for the treatment of eczema, and it currently consists of just two drugs:

- pimecrolimus (a cream, Elidel®)
- tacrolimus (an ointment, Protopic®).

At the moment, NICE recommends that only doctors with a specialist interest in skin conditions (this can include GPs) should initiate treatment with pimecrolimus or tacrolimus. They are not 'first choice' drugs (corticosteroids are tried first for treating flare ups of symptoms), and are not recommended for the treatment of the mildest cases of eczema. However, many people whose eczema has not cleared up sufficiently with corticosteroid treatment have then shown good improvements when prescribed topical immunomodulators. They have the advantage that they do not seem to cause the side-effects that can occur with long-term use of potent corticosteroids.

These drugs are fairly new, and doctors don't yet have a lot of experience with them. The limitations imposed on prescribing tacrolimus and pimecrolimus are in place to prevent putting people at risk whilst longer-term studies are carried out. These stipulate that the drugs should only be used:

- in children over the age of 2 years and adults
- for a short time only and not continuously
- in the smallest quantities that are effective.

Antihistamines and antipruritics

The doctor may prescribe antihistamine drugs in order to help relieve the itch of eczema. There is limited evidence that this treatment is effective for itch. However, as certain antihistamines may cause drowsiness in some people, they may be prescribed to help you sleep if your eczema is making this difficult.

As we saw earlier, the other drugs which the doctor may prescribe for reducing itch are called antipruritics. The most common of these drugs used in eczema are crotamiton (Eurax®, also available combined with the topical corticosteroid hydrocortisone as Eurax Hc®) and doxepin (Xepin®).

Ichthammol is also available for reducing itch in eczema, often as a paste impregnated into bandages, but is rarely used these days.

THE 'SEDATING' ANTIHISTAMINES

Generic name	Brand name(s)
Alimemazine tartrate	Vallergan®
Chlorphenamine maleate	Piriton®
Clemastine	Tavegil®
Cyproheptadine hydrochloride	Periactin®
Diphenhydramine hydrochloride	Dreemon®, Medinex®, Night-calm®, Nytol®, Panadol Night®
Hydroxyzine hydrochloride	Atarax®, Ucerax®
Promethazine hydrochloride	Phenergan®

Antibacterial, antifungal, antiviral and antibiotic drugs

Your doctor might prescribe one of these drugs (collectively known as antimicrobials) if your skin has become infected. As we have already seen, there are many topical corticosteroids and some emollients which contain antimicrobials, so these can sometimes be used to 'kill two birds with one stone'. You will usually only be prescribed these combination drugs until your infection has cleared up. Once you have completed your course you will return to your usual steroidal treatment. This is because the excessive use of antibiotics can mean that you develop resistance to them, which may

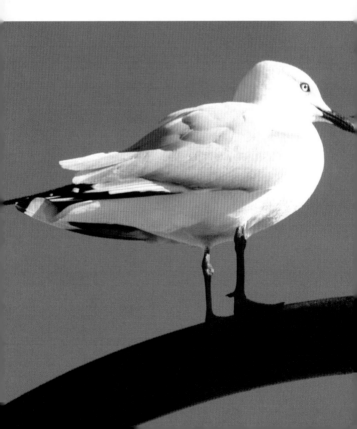

render them useless in the future. Make sure you know how long you should use antimicrobial creams or take oral antibiotics for, as it is important that you finish the course.

Usually these drugs are applied directly to the skin. However, if the infection is quite resistant, or is spread across quite a large area of your body, your doctor may decide that in order to clear up the infection it would be best for you to take a course of antibiotic tablets. If you are taking antibiotics, make sure you are aware of all the possible interactions these can have with other medicines. Antibiotics may make the oral contraceptive pill less effective, for example.

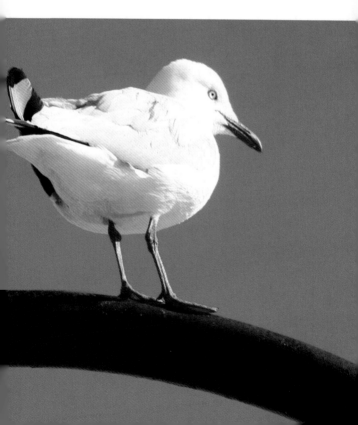

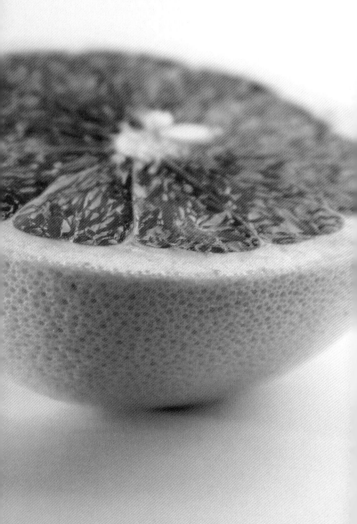

Systemic immunosuppressants

If your eczema is very severe, you might be prescribed ciclosporin by a dermatologist. Essentially, this drug acts in the same way as the topical immunomodulators, pimecrolimus and tacrolimus, by suppressing the immune response which leads to inflammation in the skin. The difference is that it is taken as a tablet, and so affects the whole body rather than just the area of skin that is affected. As it is a very potent drug with potential side-effects, it is taken for only 8 weeks at a time. It is generally used only for eczema which does not respond to any other form of treatment. More often it is given to people who have had organ transplants, to suppress the activity of their immune system and reduce the risk of the organ being rejected.

If you are taking ciclosporin, you need to be careful about exposing your skin to the sun, because it may become more susceptible to developing skin cancer. You will also be at higher risk of infections, as your immune system will be less able to fight off bacteria and viruses. It is important to inform your doctor if you think you are getting an infection or begin to feel unwell. You should avoid foods that are high in potassium, such as bananas and dried fruit, as ciclosporin can increase the concentration of potassium in your blood. You will also need to avoid grapefruit and grapefruit juice for at least an hour either side of taking a ciclosporin tablet, as they can interfere with the drug's action. The most common side-effects of ciclosporin are problems with the kidneys, high blood pressure and tremor.

Phototherapy

Phototherapy is not a treatment often used for eczema, but your specialist may consider it if your eczema is resistant to other treatments and is fairly widespread across your body.

The word phototherapy literally means light treatment. It involves standing in a booth which contains lots of light tubes that are giving out UV light. Two types of UV light are used for phototherapy – UVA and UVB, although sometimes a combination of the two is chosen. UV light is thought to benefit some people with extensive eczema because it affects the immune response in the skin which causes inflammation, in a similar manner to topical immunomodulators and ciclosporin. Because UVA light has less energy than UVB, it is often used in combination with a chemical called a psoralen. During this treatment, which is known as PUVA, the psoralen is activated by the UV light. It is the activated chemical which actually suppresses the immune response, rather than the light itself.

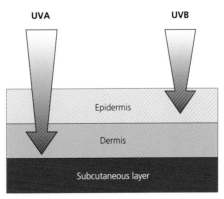

UVA LIGHT PENETRATES DEEPER INTO THE SKIN, REACHING THE DERMIS LAYER. UVB LIGHT ONLY GETS AS FAR AS THE EPIDERMIS.

If you receive phototherapy treatment, it will be administered by a dermatology nurse in a hospital, overseen by a specialist dermatologist. A course of phototherapy treatment may involve around 30 visits over the course of a few months.

The amount of UV light that your skin is exposed to must be very tightly regulated. The biggest risk associated with phototherapy is that of sunburn-like reactions. To minimise the risk of these, the nurse should also make sure that you:

- stand in the booth in the same position each time

- do not have your hair cut or change your hair style significantly between treatments

- wear goggles in the booth

- cover your genitalia if you are male.

- are not starting any new tablets that might make you sensitive to the light.

In the short-term, you can expect that phototherapy may actually aggravate itching, and can also cause tanning and dry skin. In the longer-term, there is a risk that your skin might appear to age a little faster, forming wrinkles and brown 'liver spots'. There is a small risk of skin cancer, but the amount of UV used to treat you should be low enough for this risk to be negligible.

Do NOT try to conduct your own DIY phototherapy. A sun bed is not a safe alternative to a phototherapy booth, and the treatment should only be done under close medical supervision.

TREATMENTS YOU CAN TRY YOURSELF

There is a wide range of 'natural' treatments for eczema which you can try yourself without needing a prescription from your doctor. Although you do not need your doctor's permission to try these products, it is a good idea to discuss any treatment you wish to try with your doctor first, as there may be specific reasons why certain treatments are not advisable for you to use.

Probiotics

Probiotics are basically sources of 'good bacteria'. They are made up of non-disease causing 'bugs' which are naturally found in our digestive systems. Earlier, we explored the 'hygiene hypothesis', which claims that the lack of exposure to infections in early childhood alters the way in which children's immune systems develop.

A feature of this altered immune system is a lack of good bacteria in the gut. The idea behind using probiotics for eczema is to restore these bacteria and help get the immune system working as it should – and that means fewer allergic responses.

Probiotics are found in cultured or fermented foods such as cheeses or live yoghurts, but also in supplements, which can be taken in tablets or capsules, or as an ingredient in yoghurt drinks. There are certain probiotic products which are made specifically for children. In fact, it is in young children that the strongest evidence is available supporting the use of probiotics for eczema.

Some research has indicated that giving probiotics to pregnant mothers and newborn babies might even halve the risk of the child developing eczema in the first couple of years of life. However, you should seek your doctor's advice before considering starting such a treatment in a young child.

There are no reported side-effects associated with probiotics, but it can be quite difficult to know exactly what and how much you are getting. If you are unsure as to whether it is a good idea for you to try probiotics, ask your doctor for advice.

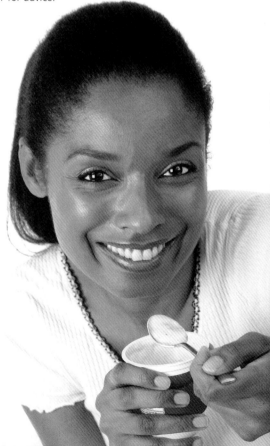

Evening primrose oil

It is thought that taking evening primrose oil may top up the levels of essential fatty acids in your body. This, as we saw earlier, can be good for restoring the suppleness and barrier function of your skin. However, there is no conclusive evidence that evening primrose oil is actually effective in eczema. Indeed, two drugs which used to be available for the treatment of eczema and contained the same active ingredient as evening primrose oil (gamolenic acid), have since been withdrawn because there was no strong evidence that they were helping people.

This is not to say, though, that evening primrose oil cannot help if you have eczema. Different treatments work for different people, so it might be worth a try! It is available from health food shops and supermarkets. If after a few months you have not seen any benefit, it is probably not worth continuing to take evening primrose oil.

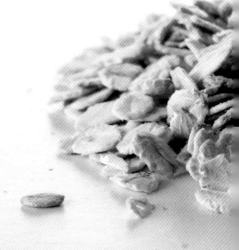

Oatmeal

Oatmeal, when applied to the skin, is thought to help relieve the itching of eczema. Many people claim that they find using oatmeal products when bathing is good for softening their skin. If you want to try oatmeal, though, don't be concerned about having to bathe in porridge! The Aveeno® range of emollient products, which includes a bath oil, contain colloidal oatmeal (an extract from oatmeal grain). Some people like to run their tap water through oatmeal grain before bathing in it.

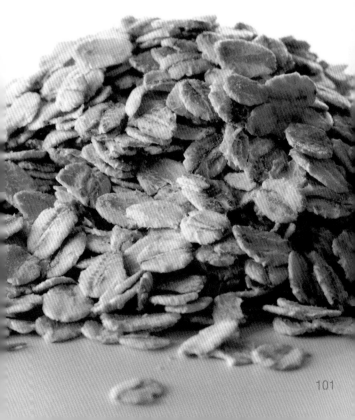

COMPLEMENTARY AND ALTERNATIVE THERAPIES

Many people use complementary treatment as part of their eczema management strategy. There are various strands of complementary medicine which are claimed to be of benefit in treating skin conditions. Unfortunately, most of them have not been tested in rigorous clinical trials in the same way as drug treatments. This means that we are less sure of how effective, or indeed, how safe, they really are.

If you wish to try complementary therapies, it is best to inform your doctor, as some herbs and other treatments may interact with the conventional medicines they are prescribing for you. Despite this, GPs are increasingly supportive of complementary medicine, and they may be able to recommend approved complementary therapists. You can also get information from societies and associations dedicated to individual therapies (see *Simple extras* page 121). Remember, though, that complementary medicine, by definition, should complement more conventional treatment strategies, not replace them altogether.

There are many complementary therapies available, but we will look at a few of those more commonly used in eczema here.

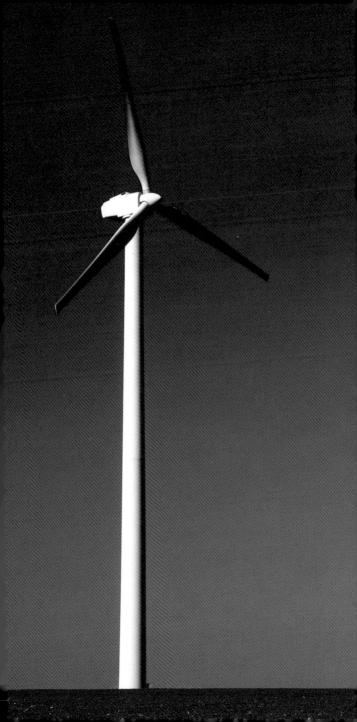

Traditional Chinese medicine

Traditional Chinese medicine uses acupuncture, blends of herbs, dietary manipulation and Tai Chi exercise to achieve balance of body, mind and environment. It is popular amongst people with eczema. It is difficult to assess formally how effective these treatments are, because there are no standard recommended doses and blends of herbs are tailored individually to each patient.

The other problem with the lack of regulation of the content of these mixtures is that sometimes, they appear to have been contaminated with traces of metals or drugs. Some forms of traditional Chinese medicine might be dangerous if you are pregnant or have liver or heart disease.

Reflexology

Reflexology involves applying manual pressure to regions of the foot, and less often the hands. It is based on the belief that all parts of the body are said to be reflected in the feet and hands.

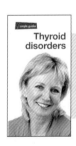

Thyroid
disorders

For more information see
Thyroid disorders

Reflexologists claim that crystalline deposits of waste products from the rest of the body collect in the foot. By working on a particular point where crystals have collected, the therapist aims to heal the corresponding area of the body. A treatment might last up to an hour, and a number of weekly sessions might be recommended. You should not have reflexology treatment if you are in the first 3 months of pregnancy, have diabetes, a thyroid disorder or any other long-term health problem.

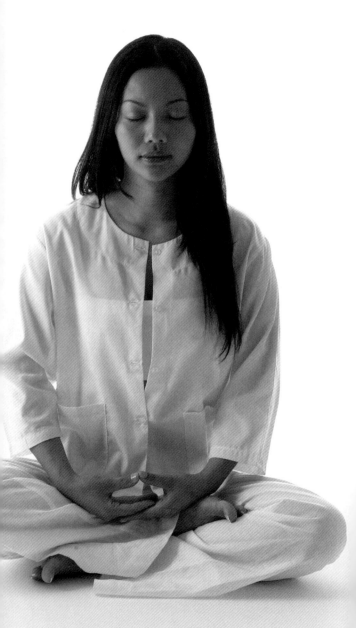

Hypnotherapy

Hypnotherapy involves being put into a relaxed hypnotic trance, during which your conscious mind can be bypassed and your subconscious mind reached. The hypnotherapist generally uses a combination of relaxation and visualisation techniques to help improve your condition. Eczema is thought to be quite susceptible to improvement with hypnotherapy. There is always a risk that hypnotherapy can make underlying psychological problems worse, so it is important that you see a properly trained practitioner. Ask your GP for advice, as he or she should be able to refer you to an NHS psychologist who practices hypnotherapy.

Acupuncture

Acupuncture is actually a part of traditional Chinese medicine, but is much better accepted in the UK than Chinese herbal therapy. By inserting fine needles into specific points on your skin, the acupuncturist aims to stimulate the flow of 'vital energy' around the body. You can expect a series of appointments, with up to 12 needles inserted at any one time. The skin pricks should not be painful, but might give you a dull, aching sensation.

The effectiveness of acupuncture for some conditions is quite well accepted, and in some areas it is even offered by the NHS. Many acupuncturists are medically qualified, so it is worth asking your doctor if you would like to try acupuncture as he or she may be able to refer you.

Homeopathy

The idea behind homeopathy is that 'like cures like'. An agent which causes relevant symptoms in a healthy individual is then given to a patient in a hugely diluted form. The treatments used are so weak that you could argue that they would be completely ineffective. A homeopathist, however, believes that it is the vibrational energy of the treatment, rather than the actual chemical content, which has the effects. After an initial consultation, you will be given your treatment in the form of tablets, granules, powders or liquid. Homeopathy is one of the better established complementary therapies in the UK, and indeed many of the therapists are actually medically qualified.

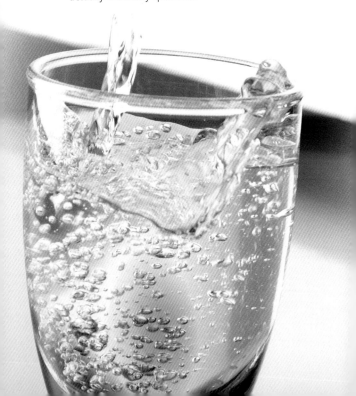

MANAGING ECZEMA IN THE ELDERLY

As we get older, our skin becomes thinner and more fragile, causing it to be susceptible to cracking and infection. If your eczema has continued into your later years, you should be particularly diligent with your application of emollients, to ensure that your skin remains as supple and strong as possible. Emollient bath oils are a useful way of moisturising your skin, and are particularly handy if you have problems with mobility and find it physically draining to apply emollient creams or lotions on a regular basis. Be aware, though, that bath oils can make a bath slippery, and you may wish to use a non-slip mat or have bath handles fitted.

Corticosteroids can be used in elderly people. However, because corticosteroids can cause the skin to thin if they are used for long periods of time, and considering the natural deterioration of skin with age, it is advisable to be particularly careful about minimising the strength and duration of corticosteroid treatment.

Older people often have smaller appetites, and eat less. It is important to keep eating well, and if you have eczema, to keep eating the particular food types that provide you with essential fatty acids. Ask your doctor for dietary supplements if you don't feel like you are getting enough of the important nutrients. You must also keep drinking plenty of fluids, to keep your skin supple and strong.

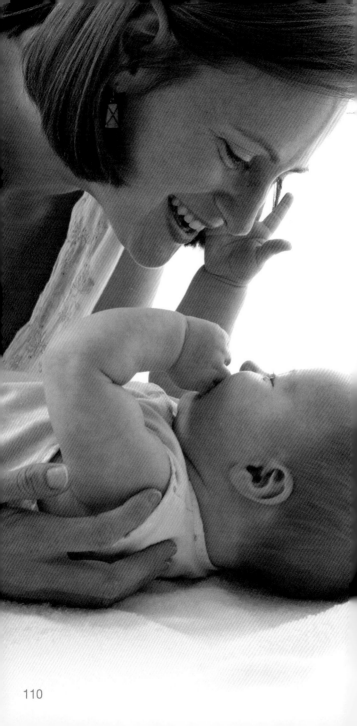

MANAGING ECZEMA DURING PREGNANCY

Some women with eczema find that their skin clears up during pregnancy whereas others find that their eczema gets worse. The treatment of eczema during pregnancy is not changed dramatically from that under normal circumstances, but the focus is shifted onto the use of emollients and avoidance of irritants and allergens that trigger flare ups. Topical corticosteroids can still be used, but usually in smaller amounts.

If you have any concerns, speak to your doctor about how much and how often you should be using corticosteroids. Certain treatments for eczema, such as some antibiotics and topical immunomodulators, should not be used during pregnancy as there is insufficient evidence that they are harmless to the unborn child.

BREAST-FEEDING AND ECZEMA

Breast-feeding is generally recommended as the best option for any newborn baby, and there is some evidence to suggest that it might protect against the development of allergies.

Some experts have claimed that prolonged breast-feeding, for at least 6 months, might be beneficial for babies at particularly high risk of atopy (e.g. if both parents and at least one sibling are atopic). However, the current evidence for this is not particularly convincing, and there have actually been reports that, rather than reducing the risk of eczema, extended breast-feeding might actually increase it.

If you are concerned about whether or not to breast-feed your child, speak to your doctor.

MANAGING OTHER FORMS OF ECZEMA

Contact eczema

The most important aspect of managing both allergic and irritant contact eczema is avoiding the trigger allergens and irritants. Identifying what these factors are can be the most difficult part of the management plan. If your doctor suspects contact eczema, he or she can arrange for you to have patch testing, where common allergens are applied to a patch of the skin, usually on your back, to assess your reaction. Typical substances which might be tested include hairdressing and dental products, plastics and glues, cosmetics and plant extracts. Your sensitivity to light might also be tested in this way.

Even when an allergen or irritant has been identified, avoiding it completely is usually not straightforward. Using gloves to protect your hands and eliminating triggers from your diet (e.g. nickel) are two possible approaches. When contact eczema is triggered, it is treated in the same way as atopic eczema.

Discoid eczema

This is treated in the much same way as atopic eczema, with emollients and topical corticosteroids the 'first choice' treatments, and antimicrobials used where infection is a problem. Oral corticosteroids, antihistamines, immunomodulating therapies and phototherapy are all available if the first choice treatments are not effective.

Seborrhoeic eczema

In many cases, this simply appears as a mild dandruff, which can be treated using a medicated shampoo (e.g. Neutrogena T-Gel® shampoo). More severe cases are treated using a combination of antimicrobials and mild topical corticosteroids (e.g. Daktacort®). Seborrhoeic eczema does tend to return periodically, but is usually fairly easy to control given proper medical attention.

Varicose eczema

This is treated primarily with emollients and, if required, topical corticosteroids. Support hosiery or bandages may be recommended to help improve circulation in the legs. Gentle exercise will also help in this respect. Varicose eczema can occur in elderly people, and so care needs to be taken not to use too much corticosteroid in these patients (see *Managing eczema in the elderly* page 109).

THE LONG AND SHORT OF IT

What does it mean for me?

Eczema is not a life-threatening illness, except very rarely, in the most severe cases. That doesn't mean that it can't be serious though. Anyone with eczema knows that eczema can be a burden, and you need to be prepared for the physical and mental impact that it may have on your life. The important thing is to be positive about it, and make sure that you feel in control of your eczema, not the other way around. You will need plenty of willpower to take good, daily care of your skin, and to avoid the things that trigger your eczema as best you can.

Will it go away?

If you have a child with eczema, remember that there is roughly a 75% chance that their symptoms will have pretty much gone away by the time they reach adulthood. Unfortunately, though, we have to leave that to Mother Nature because there is no treatment at present that can cure eczema. Some people will be troubled throughout their life by the condition.

There are a huge number of treatments available, however, and the recent emergence of the topical immunomodulators is proof that work is still being done to find better, safer medicines for eczema. By working with your doctor, you should be able to find a management plan which works for you. Whilst it may not cure your eczema, it should keep it under control.

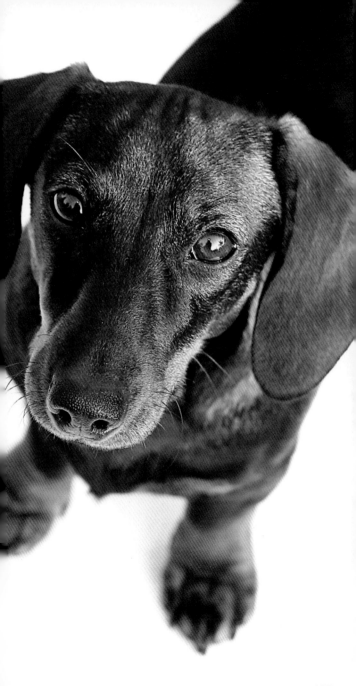

GETTING THE MOST OUT OF YOUR HEALTH SERVICE

Eczema is a long-term condition and it is important that you work together with your doctor to optimise your care. Maintaining a good relationship with your GP, specialist or any other healthcare member you may come into contact with, is fundamental to managing your eczema effectively. These people will be able to explain to you why you have eczema, why certain things can make your eczema worse, and recommend the best way to manage your symptoms. It is important that you remain in regular contact with your GP, and keep them informed of any improvement or deterioration in your symptoms. Remember, if one management approach fails to work, there are many others that can be tried.

- Don't be afraid to ask for help or advice.

- Keep your doctor informed of all the treatments you are taking, including dietary supplements.

- Know what to expect and when to ask for help.

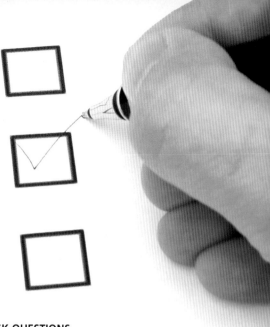

ASK QUESTIONS

Having a doctor's appointment or going to the hospital for tests can be quite a daunting prospect. It is often helpful to write down a list of questions before you attend your appointment.

- What type of eczema do I have?

- How severe is my eczema?

- It is likely to get worse?

- Do I need to have any tests?

- What type of treatment suits me best?

- What should I do if the treatment doesn't make me feel better?

- Are there any alternative or complementary therapies that might help?

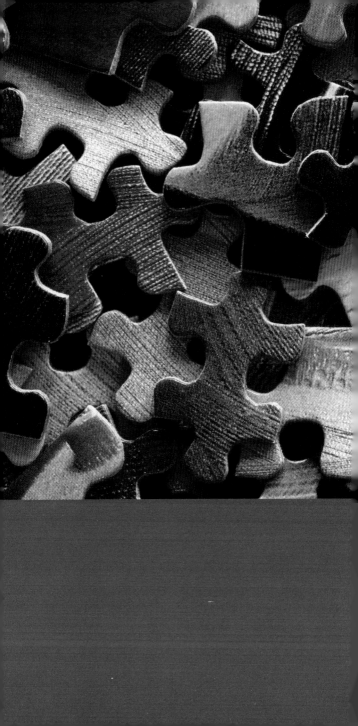

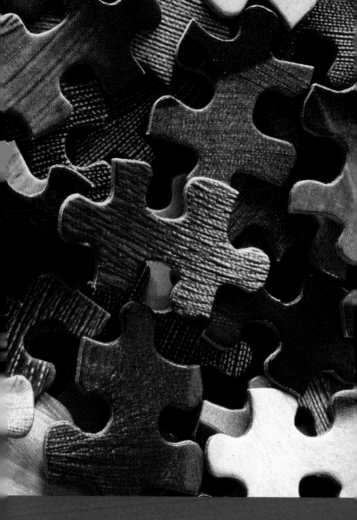

Simple
extras

FURTHER READING

■ ***BESTMEDICINE Atopic Eczema***
CSF Medical Communications Ltd, 2005
ISBN: 1-905064-95-0, £13.95
www.bestmedicine.com

■ ***BESTMEDICINE Asthma***
CSF Medical Communications Ltd, 2005
ISBN: 1-905064-94-2, £13.95
www.bestmedicine.com

■ ***Asthma (Simple Guide)***
CSF Medical Communications Ltd, 2005
ISBN: 1-905466-00-5, £5.99
www.bestmedicine.com

■ ***Thyroid disorders (Simple Guide)***
CSF Medical Communications Ltd, 2006
ISBN: 1-905466-09-9, £5.99
www.bestmedicine.com

■ **Guidelines for the management of atopic eczema**
Primary Care Dermatology Society and British
Association of Dermatologists.
www.bad.org.uk

■ **Prodigy Guidance – Eczema – atopic**
www.prodigy.nhs.uk

■ **Prodigy Guidance – Dermatitis – contact**
www.prodigy.nhs.uk

USEFUL CONTACTS

▨ **Association of Reflexologists**
27 Old Gloucester Road
London
WC1N 3XX
Tel: 0870 5673320
Email: *info@aor.org.uk*
Website: *www.aor.org.uk*

▨ **British Acupuncture Council (BAcC)**
63 Jeddo Road
London
W12 9HQ
Tel: 020 8735 0400
Email: *info@acupuncture.org.uk*
Website: *www.acupuncture.org.uk*

▨ **British Association of Dermatologists**
4 Fitzroy Square
London
WIT 5HQ
Tel: 0207 3830266
Email: *admin@bad.org.uk*
Website: *www.bad.org.uk*

▨ **British Homeopathic Association (BHA)**
Hahnemann House
29 Park Street West
Luton
LU1 3BE
Tel: 0870 4443950
Website: *www.trusthomeopathy.org*

■ **British Medical Acupuncture Society (BMAS)**
BMAS House
3 Winnington Court
Northwich
CW8 1AQ
Tel: 01606 786782
Email: *admin@medical-acupuncture.org.uk*
Website: *www.medical-acupuncture.co.uk*

■ **British Society of Medical and Dental Hypnosis**
28 Dale Park Gardens
Cookridge
Leeds
LS16 7PJ
Tel: 07000 560309
Email: *nat.office@bsmdh.org*
Website: *www.bsmdh.org*

■ **Eczema Voice**
PO Box 5448
Milton Keynes
MK4 1XJ
Website: *www.eczemavoice.com*

■ **National Council for Hypnotherapy**
PO Box 421
Charwelton
Daventry
NN11 1AS
Tel: 0800 9520545
Website: *www.hypnotherapists.org.uk*

National Eczema Society
Hill House
Highgate Hill
London
N19 5NA
Helpline: 0870 2413604
Email: *helpline@eczema.org*
Website: *www.eczema.org*

National Institute for Health and Clinical Excellence (NICE)
11 The Strand
London
WC2N 5HR
Tel: 020 7766 9191
Website: *www.nice.org.uk*

NHS Direct
NHS Direct Line: 0845 46 47
Website: *www.nhsdirect.nhs.uk*

Primary Care Dermatology Society
Gable House
40 High Street
Rickmansworth
Herts
WD3 1ER
Tel: 01923 711678
Email: *pcds@pcds.org.uk*
Website: *www.pcds.org.uk*

■ **The Acupuncture Society**
27 Cavendish Drive
Edgware
Middlesex
HA8 7NR
Tel: 0773 4668402
Email: *acupuncturesocietyuk@yahoo.co.uk*
Website: *www.acupuncturesociety.org.uk*

■ **The British Institute of Homeopathy**
Cygnet House
Market Square
Staines
Middlesex
TW18 4RH
Tel: 01784 440467
Email: *info@britinsthom.com*
Website: *www.britinsthom.com*

■ **The British Reflexology Association**
Monks Orchard
Whitbourne
Worcester
WR6 5RB
Tel: 01886 821207
Email: *bra@britreflex.co.uk*
Website: *www.britreflex.co.uk*

■ **The National Register of Hypnotherapists and Psychotherapists (NRHP)**
12 Cross Street
Nelson
BB9 7EN
Helpline: 0800 1613823
Email: *nrhp@btconnect.com*
Website *www.nrhp.co.uk*

■ **The Register of Chinese Herbal Medicine**
Website: *www.rchm.co.uk*

■ **The Skin Care Campaign**
Website: *www.skincarecampaign.org*

YOUR RIGHTS

As a patient, you have a number of important rights. These include the right to the best possible standard of care, the right to information, the right to dignity and respect, the right to confidentiality and underpinning all of these, the right to good health.

Occasionally, you may feel as though your rights have been compromised, or you may be unsure of where you stand when it comes to qualifying for certain treatments or services. In these instances, there are a number of organisations you can turn to for help and advice. Remember that lodging a complaint against your health service should not compromise the quality of care you receive, either now or in the future.

■ **The Patients Association**
The Patients Association (*www.patients-association.com*) is a UK charity which represents patient rights, influences health policy and campaigns for better patient care.
Contact details:
PO Box 935
Harrow
Middlesex
HA1 3YJ
Helpline: 0845 6084455
Email: *mailbox@patients-association.com*

■ **Citizens Advice Bureau**
The Citizens Advice Bureau (*www.nacab.org.uk*) provides free, independent and confidential advice to NHS patients at a number of outreach centres located throughout the country (*www.adviceguide.org.uk*).
Contact details:
Find your local Citizens Advice Bureau using the search tool at *www.citizensadvice.org.uk*.

■ **Patient Advice and Liaison Services (PALS)**

Set up by the Department of Health (*www.dh.gov.uk*), PALS provide information, support and confidential advice to patients, families and their carers.

Contact details:

Phone your local hospital, clinic, GP surgery or health centre and ask for details of the PALS, or call NHS Direct on 0845 46 47.

■ **The Independent Complaints Advocacy Service (ICAS)**

ICAS is an independent service that can help you bring about formal complaints against your NHS practitioner. ICAS provides support, help, advice and advocacy from experienced advisors and caseworkers.

Contact details:

ICAS Central Team

Myddelton House

115–123 Pentonville Road

London N1 9LZ

Email: *icascentralteam@citizensadvice.org.uk*

Or contact your local ICAS office direct.

Accessing your medical records

You have a legal right to see all your health records under the Data Protection Act of 1998. You can usually make an informal request to your doctor and you should be given access within 40 days. Note that you may have to pay a small fee for the privilege.

You can be denied access to your records if your doctor believes that the information contained within them could cause serious harm to you or another person. If you are applying for access on behalf of someone else, then you will not be granted access to information which the patient gave to his or her doctor on the understanding that it would remain confidential.

PERSONAL RECORD:

My Simple Guide

This Simple Guide belongs to:

Name:

Address:

Tel:

Email:

In case of emergency please contact:

Name:

Address:

Tel:

Email:

My Healthcare Team

GP surgery address and telephone number

Name:

Address:

Tel:

I am registered with Dr

My dermatology nurse

My dermatologist

Other members of my healthcare team

NOTES

NOTES

NOTES

NOTES

NOTES

NOTES

NOTES

SIMPLE GUIDE QUESTIONNAIRE

Dear reader,

We would love to know what you thought of this Simple Guide. Please take a few moments to fill out this short questionnaire and return it to us at the FREEPOST address below.

CSF Medical Communications Ltd
FREEPOST NAT5703
Witney
OX29 8BR

SO WHAT DID YOU THINK?

Which Simple Guide have you just read?

_____

Where did you buy it (store/town)?

_____

Who did you buy it for?

☐ Myself ☐ Friend ☐ Relative
☐ Patient ☐ Other

Where did you hear about the Simple Guides?

☐ They were recommended to me ☐ Internet
☐ Stumbled across them ☐ Other

Did it meet with your expectations?

☐ Exceeded ☐ Met all
☐ Met most ☐ Fell below

Was there anything you particularly liked?

_____

_____

_____

Was there anything we could have improved?

_____

_____

_____

WHO ARE YOU?

Name: _____

Address: _____

_____

_____

Tel: _____

Email: _____

How old are you?
☐ Under 25   ☐ 25–34   ☐ 35–44
☐ 45–54   ☐ 55–64   ☐ 65+

Are you...   ☐ Male   ☐ Female

Do you suffer from a long-term medical condition? If so, please specify.

_____

WHAT NEXT?

What other topics would you like to see covered in future Simple Guides?

Thanks,
the Simple Guides team